TREATING DIGESTIVE DISORDERS FROM AN ENDOBIOGENIC PERSPECTIVE

An Innovative System of Plant Medicine

Paul Michael

AEON

First published in 2021 by
Aeon Books
PO Box 76401
London W5 9RG

British Library Cataloguing in Publication Data

A C.I.P. for this book is available from the British Library

ISBN-13: 978-1-91159-755-1

Typeset by Medlar Publishing Solutions Pvt Ltd, India
Printed in Great Britain

www.aeonbooks.co.uk

CONTENTS

Paul Michael is a medical herbalist, practitioner of endobiogenic medicine and a qualified Gut and Psychology Syndrome (GAPS) therapist. He is a first-class graduate of the BSc in Herbal Medicine programme at Middlesex University, and a member of one of the main professional organisations for medical herbalists in the UK, the College of Practitioners of Phytotherapy (CPP). He has trained for over 7 years with Dr Jean-Claude Lapraz, and in his practice uses the endobiogenic approach in conjunction with classical herbal medicine. Paul Michael has written articles for *Positive Health Magazine*, and has hosted a series of radio talk shows focusing on the approach of modern herbal medicine in the treatment of disease. Paul has been involved in the teaching of endobiogenic medicine in the UK and is one of the founders of the Endobiogenic Medicine Society of the UK (EMS).

Paul has first-hand experience of inflammatory bowel disease (IBD) as he was diagnosed with Crohn's disease at the age of 19. He was never happy with the thought of taking conventional medication for Crohn's disease and was determined to find another way. It was this personal experience and determination that led him eventually to study phytotherapy; he is passionate about helping others with chronic illness so that they do not have to suffer needlessly.

Paul has been in remission from Crohn's for 18 years using phytotherapy and diet. Paul has also trained in the traditional Chinese internal healing arts of Qigong and Tai Chi and has a very strong interest in mind–body medicine.

FOREWORD

This new book by Paul Michael brings together three areas that have long fascinated me as a medical herbalist and healthcare practitioner: the workings of the digestive system, and its profound influence on general health; the extraordinary healing capacity of medicinal plants; and endobiogenic medicine—first formulated in France by Drs Christian Duraffourd and Jean-Claude Lapraz—which I have studied for well on 30 years.

Since training with me on the Herbal Medicine BSc at Middlesex University, Paul has worked single-mindedly on developing his expertise in endobiogenic medicine, both by rigorously applying it in his professional practice and by training with the two foremost exponents of endobiogeny in the world today, Drs Jean-Claude Lapraz and Dr Kamyar Hedayat. Indeed, he is one of the very few practitioners in the UK to have gained a qualification in endobiogeny with the Systems Biology Research Group co-chaired by Drs Lapraz and Hedayat.

The term endobiogeny will no doubt be unfamiliar to most English-speaking readers, but in this book Paul explains, with great clarity, its underlying principles and practical applications in medicine, illustrating these with vivid case histories from his own practice. His focus is, of course, digestive disorders, which, as well as being one of the commonest presentations in practice, also has a profound personal meaning for Paul. Since he is also a qualified GAPS therapist, he has a keen interest in the therapeutic potential of certain dietary regimes, for example, in IBD. Diet is, of course, combined with herbal medicine, which is one of the key agents of endobiogenic therapy.

Again, Paul devotes considerable attention to novel approaches to treating abdominal adhesions (which are common in the many IBD patients who have undergone abdominal surgery), including manual therapy and specific exercises.

This book, then, will be of interest to all those who seek and study integrative approaches to disease, and particularly to disease involving the digestive tract. I am convinced that they will be impressed by the outstanding results practitioners can get by adopting a genuine systems approach that targets the root cause of digestive (and other) imbalances, and uses plant medicines in a totally new way to restore equilibrium.

Colin Nicholls
President
Endobiogenic Medicine Society UK

ACKNOWLEDGEMENTS

I believe that it is important to give acknowledgement and thanks for the work undertaken in the past and the knowledge and experience shared.

I would like to thank Colin Nicholls (President of EMS), who was one of my lecturers at Middlesex University when I was studying phytotherapy, and was the person who introduced me to endobiogenic medicine and to Dr Jean-Claude Lapraz. In fact, he was the one who first introduced the UK to endobiogenic medicine. Colin has been a great help over the years, and is a person of great integrity who is always willing to provide support and guidance.

I would also like to thank Dr Lapraz, my mentor, a most modest and extraordinarily intelligent person. I have known Dr Lapraz for about 18 years now and I always look forward to seeing him and learning from him. He is always ready to share his immense knowledge with his students. I am indebted to him both for his invaluable help in stabilising my own medical condition and for his guidance and tuition in the field of endobiogeny.

Thanks, are also due to Dr Kamyar Hedayat for his profound work in the development of endobiogenic medicine.

Above all, thanks to my family for all their support during the writing of this book, and to all the others who contributed by way of interview or the sharing of knowledge. If it were not for all these people, this book would not have been possible.

For all of this, I am truly grateful.

INTRODUCTION

What is endobiogenic medicine (endobiogeny)?

Endobiogeny is a theory of terrain that assesses how the internal life of the body is generated and sustained.

Endobiogeny

Endo—meaning *internal*

Bio—meaning *life*

Geny—meaning *origin*

The terms endobiogeny and endobiogenic thus refer to the origins of internal life.

Christian Duraffourd MD conceived the endobiogenic concept, and its teaching was developed by Drs Christian Duraffourd and Jean-Claude Lapraz. Drs Duraffourd and Lapraz decided very early on to use plant medicines as the treatment modality as the complexity of the plants perfectly match the complexity of the human organism.

Endobiogenic medicine is a system of medicine that considers the endocrine system to be the true manager of the body. It is the true manager, as it is the only system that manages itself and every other system in the body. The autonomic nervous system helps to regulate the endocrine system. It regulates the intensity and duration of the endocrine function.

The theory of terrain is principal to the endobiogenic concept. When we speak about terrain, we mean the internal environment of the body. The environment of the cells, the tissues and the organs and how these function as a whole.

To explain the terrain: in my clinic, I use the analogy of a house that has mould growing in it. In order for mould to grow, there needs to be a suitable environment (terrain) for the spores to take root. If you simply use mould killer and clean the mould, it will keep coming back. You need to address the reason why the mould is there in the first place. Why is the environment suitable for the mould to survive and flourish? Once you change the environment of the house, e.g. stop drying your clothes on the radiators, add an extractor in the kitchen, install a positive air system etc. the mould will no longer find a home.

If we look at recurrent infection, we can see this theory at play in the human body. Have you ever wondered why some people are prone to specific infections and others are not? If we simply use anti-infectious agents, we may not succeed in preventing recurrent infection from returning or we may have to use anti-infectious agents constantly. On the other hand, if we alter the environment within, the infectious agent, whether it be a bacteria, virus or fungus, will not be able to grow and become pathogenic.

During the course of this book we will look closely at how the endocrine and autonomic nervous systems effect the terrain; specifically, in relation to the digestive system. We will look at treatment modalities, from an endobiogenic perspective, that alter the terrain in a positive way. Several detailed case studies will be presented, allowing you to see how patients are treated within this model of medicine. We will also discuss the functional biology (unique blood test) used to identify imbalances and to track patient progress. The functional biology shows over 150 markers and is unlike any other blood test.

CHAPTER ONE

The terrain

Before we focus on the digestive system we must first look, in detail, at the autonomic nervous system and then at the endocrine system in order to understand their effects globally and then specifically on the digestive system. How do these system's affect the terrain?

On the subject of the terrain

We have already touched on the concept.
     The concept of *'terrain'* is the cornerstone of endobiogenic medicine.

- The terrain is the environment within the body, within the tissues and the cells.
- The terrain is governed by the endocrine and the autonomic nervous systems.

> The germ is nothing. The terrain is everything.
>
> (*Louis Pasteur*, 1822–1895)

The environment that we talk about is linked macroscopically and microscopically, i.e. external factors and internal factors are at play.

Factors that modify the terrain:

- **Iatrogenic causes,** for example:
    - antibiotics profoundly modify the environment of the gut and can have devastating effects on the microbiome. We now know that the microbiota plays

a major role in health and disease. The microbiome of infants is especially susceptible to damage from antibiotics. Research has shown that antibiotics used in the first years of life have highly detrimental and long-lasting effects. There is a link between antibiotics used in early life and the development of disease in later life.[1]

– Nonsteroidal anti-inflammatory drugs (NSAIDs) and proton pump inhibitors (PPIs). These are two of the most commonly prescribed medications; both have severe effects on the integrity of the gastrointestinal system. Capsule endoscopy studies have shown that even low doses of NSAIDs cause damage to the gut mucosa. In addition to this, the frequent use of PPIs alongside NSAIDs has been shown to potentiate the damaging effects of NSAIDs on the gut lining. This is due to the fact that PPIs modify the microbiome of the intestine. Researchers now believe that even very minor damage to the mucosa of the intestines can have severe metabolic consequences for the patient.[2]

- **Chemical toxins**. According to a paper published by *PLOS Biology*, 'there are now over 85,000 chemicals now approved for use in commerce'.[3] Toxic chemicals have been linked to many diseases. One example is Parkinson's disease. Studies show that rotenone, an isoflavone used as a broad-spectrum insecticide and pesticide, paraquat, a herbicide and organochlorines are linked to increased risks of developing Parkinson's disease.[4]

- **Stress**. Stress is a major factor in the modification of the terrain. When we say stress, we mean any aggressor. Dr Lapraz uses this word 'aggressor' to mean anything that stresses the patient, whether it be physical, emotional, spiritual or environmental. A virus or bacteria is an aggressor. A toxin is also an aggressor. Stress causes profound changes at every level of the organism and brings into play the general syndrome of adaptation in its means to regulate body systems.

- **Puberty, andropause and menopause**. These are sensitive times in a person's life where the body is changing its function and finding a new balance. Hence, it is a critical time where things can go wrong and disease can present. Furthermore, in endobiogenic medicine there is what we call the phenomenon of recycling which occurs every 7 years. At this point the organism re-evaluates how it has been functioning and changes its function. It does not function in the same way again.

These are all factors which modify the terrain in various ways. Once the terrain is altered in a negative way, then disease can present itself, whether chronic infections, autoimmune disease or even more serious disease.

Pre-critical and critical terrain

In endobiogenic medicine there exist the phenomenon of two states of terrain. The pre-critical and the critical.

1. *The pre-critical terrain* is the terrain that exists which determines susceptibility to a condition or conditions.
2. *The critical terrain* is the state of terrain when the condition or conditions are active, i.e. in an active disease process.

For example, let's look at someone who has Crohn's disease and is in the pre-critical terrain state. This is an individual who is predisposed to having Crohn's flare-ups but is not in a state of an acute attack at present. They are not presenting with a flare-up but the terrain exists that favours this specific condition. If the right trigger/triggers are in place this individual can move from the pre-critical to the critical terrain state. Let's say this person is subjected to emotional stress for a reasonable time period. Let's say they are bullied at work for a few months. This emotional stress can induce a flare-up. They are now in the critical terrain state and in an active disease process.

On the other hand, an individual who does not have a pre-critical terrain that favours Crohn's disease will not have a flare-up of Crohn's even if they are subjected to the same emotional stress.

CHAPTER TWO

The autonomic nervous system

We will now take the time to look at how endobiogenic medicine views the role of the autonomic nervous system in relation to the disease process and its role in the management of the terrain. Before we do this lets first remind ourselves of some important basic facts about this amazing system.

What is the autonomic nervous system and what does it do?

The autonomic nervous system is the part of our nervous system that is not generally in our control. I say generally, as there are certain individuals, masters of various disciplines, throughout history, and also modern-day individuals, that have exhibited the ability to effect changes in their autonomic nervous system at will.

The autonomic nervous system (ANS) consists of visceral motor nerve fibres that regulate the activity of smooth muscles, cardiac muscles and glands. It controls functions such as, digestion, pupil constriction and dilation and heart rate (see Table 1).

Table 1. Effects of autonomic nerve activity on effector tissues[5]

Tissue	Sympathetic Receptor	Sympathetic Stimulation	Parasympathetic Stimulation
Eye			
Radial muscle of the iris	α_1	Contraction (dilation of the pupil; mydriasis)	–

(Continued)

Table 1. (Continued)

Tissue	Sympathetic Receptor	Sympathetic Stimulation	Parasympathetic Stimulation
Sphincter muscle of the iris		–	Contraction (constriction of the pupil; miosis)
Ciliary muscle	β_2	Relaxation for far vision	Contraction for near vision
Heart	β_1, β_2	↑ Heart rate	↓ Heart rate
		↑ Force of contraction	↓ Rate of conduction
		↑ Rate of conduction	
Arterioles			
Skin	α_1	Strong constriction	–
Abdominal viscera	α_1	Strong constriction	–
Kidney	α_1	Strong constriction	–
Skeletal muscle	α_1, β_2	Weak constriction	–
Spleen	α_1	Contraction	
Lungs			
Airways	β_2	Bronchodilation	Bronchoconstriction
Glands	α_1, β_2	↓ Secretion	↑ Secretion
Liver	α_1, β_2	Glycogenolysis	–
		Gluconeogenesis	–
Adipose tissue	β_3	Lipolysis	–
Sweat glands	Muscarinic	Generalised sweating	–
	α_1	Localised sweating	–
Piloerector muscles	α_1	Contraction (erection of hair, goose bumps)	–
Adrenal medullae	Nicotinic	↑ Secretion of epinephrine, norepinephrine	–
Salivary glands	α_1, β_2	Small volume K + and water secretion	Large volume K+ and water secretion; amylase secretion
Stomach			
Motility	α_1, β_2	Decreased	Increased
Sphincters	α_1	Contraction	Relaxation
Secretion			Stimulation
Intestine			
Motility	α_1, β_2	Decreased	Increased

(Continued)

Table 1. (Continued)

Tissue	Sympathetic Receptor	Sympathetic Stimulation	Parasympathetic Stimulation
Sphincters	α_1	Contraction	Relaxation
Secretion			Stimulation
Gallbladder	β_2	Relaxation	Contraction
Pancreas			
Exocrine	α	$\downarrow$ Enzyme secretion	$\uparrow$ Enzyme secretion
Endocrine (Islets B-cells)	α	$\downarrow$ Insulin secretion	$\uparrow$ Insulin secretion
Urinary bladder			
Detrusor muscle (bladder wall)	β_2	Relaxation	Contraction
Urethra sphincter		Contraction	Relaxation
Kidney	β_1	$\uparrow$ Renin secretion	–

Subdivisions of the autonomic nervous system

Typically, the autonomic nervous system consists of the following two divisions:

- **Sympathetic nervous system**—stimulated by stress states and exercise. Any kind of aggression on the body or mind, as mentioned above, stimulates the sympathetic division.
- **Parasympathetic system**—rest and digest. Relaxation.

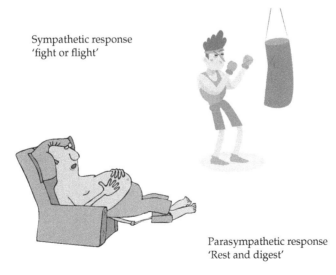

Sympathetic response 'fight or flight'

Parasympathetic response 'Rest and digest'

Figure 1. Autonomic nervous system response.

The sympathetic and parasympathetic divisions exhibit opposite effects on the same visceral organ. One can stimulate and the other can inhibit. Conventionally the autonomic nervous system is categorised into parasympathetic and sympathetic, betasympathetic is not necessarily recognised as a separate division of the autonomic nervous system, but falls under the category of sympathetic activity.

I have found that many doctors and therapists consider that having a high parasympathetic activity is good, because para equals relaxation. For this reason, they believe that stimulating para activity is beneficial. In addition, they view that having a high sympathetic state is detrimental, as it is linked to stress states. This may seem to make sense based on what we have said so far about the autonomic nervous system. However, it is not as simple as this. In reality, there is a much more intricate and dynamic activity at play.

The subject of the autonomic nervous system and its divisions (parasympathetic, alphasympathetic and betasympathetic) needs further explanation. Notice I have split the sympathetic into alpha- and betasympathetic. We will look at this in detail in the next section entitled endobiogenic medicine perspective.

A patient that has high parasympathetic activity is not a healthy person. It does not simply mean high para equals relaxation. There are negative consequences to having a high para, as is the case with any imbalance. We need to consider the relative activity between all the divisions of the autonomic nervous system and the effect on one another.

In order to clarify and understand exactly what occurs in each of these divisions, we need to break it down and look at each division separately, evaluating their effects on the body. Once we have done this, we can then put it all together and observe its combined effect, as a total system. This process will assist in understanding the implications of having imbalances in the autonomic nervous system at each level and the role these imbalances play in the development and progression of disease.

As a practitioner, if you have a clear understanding of the role that the autonomic nervous system plays in the modification of the terrain and hence disease, you will already be able to obtain very good results with a wide range of conditions, including gastrointestinal disease.

Endobiogenic medicine perspective

Endobiogenic medicine places greater emphasis on distinguishing between the divisions of the autonomic nervous system. The divisions are as follows:

- Parasympathetic
- Alphasympathetic
- Betasympathetic

The sympathetic division is clearly subdivided into alpha and beta.

In endobiogenic medicine it is essential to understand the effects of each of these divisions and subdivisions (para, alpha and beta) thoroughly, as they are intricately linked in the disease process. In response to an aggressor the ANS adjusts the internal environment of the body, and plays a major role in the modification of the terrain, as seen in Table 1. The ANS adjusts heart rate, blood pressure, body temperature and increases or decreases secretions. Fine adjustments are made all the time between para, alpha and beta.

Let's now take a look in detail at each of these systems. At the end of each section, a list will be provided of some of the important para, alpha and beta effects, signs and symptoms which may be present. They may not all be present in the patient as patients are rarely imbalanced purely in one way. There are usually multiple imbalances in the ANS when there is illness and this depends on the case. This will be explained in more depth as the chapter unfolds.

Parasympathetic

The main neurotransmitter for the parasympathetic system is acetylcholine (ACh).[6] ACh is made up of, choline plus acetyl CoA and ACh-releasing fibres are called cholinergic fibres. ACh receptors are nicotinic and muscarinic receptors though their effect differs from one another.[7]

The function of the parasympathetic nervous system

1. Anabolism. The parasympathetic system is an anabolic system, a nutritive system. It is involved in building and restoring.
2. Assimilation.

   Mainly solicited:

   - Para rises at night in order to prepare the organism for sleep.
   - During and after meals.
   - During infancy, as it is an important time of growth.

Main actions of the parasympathetic system

This is not a list of all of the actions of the parasympathetic system but rather a list of the important actions related to digestive activity in order to help build a picture of how it is implicated in specific conditions. The parasympathetic system:

- Relaxes the sphincters of the stomach and intestines.
- Increases motility of the intestines and the gall bladder.
- Increases all secretions: there are more fluids, however, they are less concentrated. For example, there is an increase in digestive secretions and choleresis.
- Has a hypoglycaemic action. This is because the vagus nerve (one of the main parasympathetic nerves) stimulates the pancreas and thereby increases insulin secretion.

Vagus nerve

The vagus nerve is the tenth cranial nerve and is the main component of the para-sympathetic nervous system. As such, it plays a major role in the maintenance of metabolic homeostasis. The vagus nerve is important in regulating the function of the intestines; it regulates the contraction of smooth muscles and stimulates glandular secretions.[8] It also has an important relationship with the pancreas, as mentioned earlier.

Vagotonia

What is vagotonia? *It is a state of autonomic nervous system dysregulation.* When vagoto-nia is present, there is a shift in the balance of the autonomic nervous system towards parasympathetic activity. There is greater parasympathetic activity relative to sympa-thetic activity.

   Important to note: insufficiency of the exocrine pancreas will stimulate para, as the organism tries to compensate for the insufficiency by stimulating more secretions. This rise in para is a co-factor in illness and must be recognised and taken into consid-eration when treating patients.

Important parasympathetic effects, signs and symptoms

- More digestive activity.
- Increased salivation.
- Increases mucus secretion.
- Plays a major role in congestion as it increases secretions.
- Low pulse, low heart rate, low blood pressure.
- Wet/damp hands and feet, sweaty.
- Greater urge to pass urine, especially at night. This is because para is higher at night.
- Post-prandial somnolence.
- Eye pupils constricted to protect eyes and lenses in the eyes set for close vision.
- Para is an anabolic state, so a high para can be linked to weight gain. It is not always the case that a patient with a high para will be overweight. It depends on many other factors as to whether the person will be in a net anabolic or a net catabolic state. This can seem to be a contradiction, but in actual fact it is not. A person can have a high para but at the same time there could be multiple endocrine imbalances that have a catabolic effect on the organism, i.e. the person will not be overweight. This will become clearer when we delve deeper into the effects of the endocrine system.

Sympathetic

To clarify again: in endobiogenic medicine there is a clear distinction between alphasympathetic and betasympathetic.

Chemical mediators:

- **Dopamine**. Dopamine is referred to in endobiogenic terms as central alpha. Later on, we will discuss the concept of central and peripheral in more detail. For now, central pertains to 'at the brain level' and peripheral pertains to 'at the body level'. So, dopamine is central alpha and rises as a result of an increase in alpha activity. Mesolimbic dopamine has been shown to rise in states of stress and trauma.[9] Dopamine and thyrotropin-releasing hormone (TRH), which is central beta, are linked to anxiety states and states of increased mental activity. We will discuss this further on.
- **Noradrenaline**. Noradrenaline in endobiogenic medicine is peripheral alpha. It is the main alphasympathetic neurotransmitter and is linked to states of excitement and stress.[10]
- **Adrenaline**. The main peripheral betasympathetic neurotransmitter. Adrenaline is responsible for the fight or flight response. This has been known for some time now. However, adrenalin has an important metabolic role with regards to the mobilisation of energy stores in the form of glucose and free fatty acids which are needed for movement. Hence beta is an active system, and it is involved in movement. Adrenalin is also needed in order for the organism to overcome hypoglycaemia.[11]

Sympathetic receptor types are adrenergic

As seen in Table 1, the two major classes of receptors are *alpha* and *beta*. Receptor subclasses are alpha1 and alpha2; beta1, beta2 and beta3. For the purpose of this book we will simply be looking at the broad terms, alpha and beta.

Alphasympathetic

The alphasympathetic system is linked to and stimulated by excitement and stress. When under stress, the organism releases noradrenaline, adrenaline, cortisol and glucagon, in order to successfully adapt to the aggression. These are catabolic hormones,[12] hence the alphasympathetic system is a catabolic system, as it mobilises energy that the organism will need to keep functioning.

The alphasympathetic system is also a constrictive system. When it is activated, there is vascular constriction at the level of the skin, kidneys, liver and spleen. There is also constriction of the bronchioles, of the muscles of the uterus and bladder and of the sphincters. For example, the sphincter of Oddi contracts and remains shut under the influence of alpha.

The alphasympathetics constrictive effect on the digestive sphincters is of paramount importance in understanding how the autonomic nervous system is affecting the GI system. In this example, we are speaking of the sphincter of Oddi. The sphincter of Oddi is a valve that controls the flow of bile and pancreatic juice that leaves the liver and pancreas and empties into the duodenum. See Figure 2. If alphasympathetic activity is very high, the sphincter of Oddi will remain shut and digestion will be impaired. Furthermore, alpha reduces the motility of the gallbladder; thus, impairing the flow of bile.

As alpha is a constrictive system it also plays a role in some forms of constipation as it reduces gut motility.

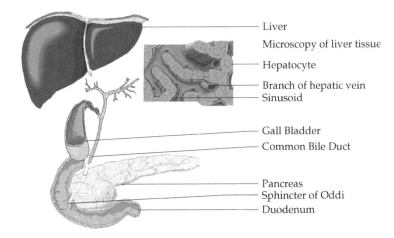

Figure 2. The sphincter of Oddi.

The function of the alphasympathetic system

1. Reactivity, especially of the senses. Patients with high alpha activity are very sensitive and very reactive people. They are hypersensitive at every level; internally to their own thoughts and to the external environment.
2. Catabolism, as mentioned above.
3. Alpha is involved in the volumetric adjustment, calibration and priming of the different secretions. This includes the hormones. Alpha plays a role in the concentration of the secretions as a constrictive system; it allows the fluids to become more concentrated.[13]

Important alphasympathetic effects, signs and symptoms

- Alpha has a hyperglycaemic action; this is prolonged and calibrated by the inhibition of insulin secretion.[13] This rise in blood glucose is essential as the brain needs an energetic substrate in order to keep functioning in times of stress. The more stress there is, the greater the energy requirement is. Patients that are unable to access stored energy in times of stress are the type of patients that need to sleep immediately after a stressful event has occurred.
- The liver is sensitive to sympathetic activity via alpha vasoconstriction, which can modify the blood flow. By so doing, it causes a modification of hepatic metabolites

(e.g. glycogenolysis and glycogenesis).[13] This is important to remember, as it is linked to congestion.
- Alpha decreases secretion levels in cells of biliary canaliculi.
- Alpha plays a major role in congestion as it is a constrictive system. Imagine a garden hose pipe: if you step on it, the water will not flow freely. It becomes restricted. This is the effect of alpha.
- Digestive activity and urinary activity reduced. Patients can present with constipation and or difficulty passing urine.
- Dry mouth.
- Cold hands and feet.
- Fast pulse, fast heart rate and high blood pressure (blood vessels constrict).
- Rapid breathing.
- Dilated pupils.
- Brain activity elevated.

This is in response to any aggressor whether physical, mental or spiritual.

Betasympathetic

The function of the betasympathetic system.

- Initially, there is a brief overactivation of the constriction started by the alphasympathetic system, followed by a discharge resulting in the relaxation of:
  1. The sphincters
  2. The muscles of the uterus and bladder
  3. The bronchi
  4. The blood vessels

Betasympathetic is the release mechanism that resets the cycle.

- Excretion of the different secretions.
- A very brief increase in all the parameters of the myocardium: frequency, excitability, conductivity; but if the duration or the frequency is increased it can create anomalies such as palpitations.[13]
- An amplification of the hyperglycaemic action which is induced by the alphasympathetic system, following, after release, a return to normal.[13] Adrenalin substantially increases blood glucose levels. It does this by increasing hepatic glucose production by stimulating glycogenolysis and gluconeogenesis and by suppressing insulin. In addition to this, the hyperglycaemic action of adrenalin is potentiated by glucagon and cortisol.[11]
- An increase in lipolysis.

For the reasons mentioned above, the function of the sympathetic system as a whole, i.e. alpha and beta are responsible for the calibration and delivery of the energetic substrates to the cells of the heart, brain and muscles.

The sympathetic system as a whole (alpha and beta) is activated mainly:

- During the day.
- When fasting.
- During puberty and menopause: puberty and menopause are particularly critical times when the organism needs to adapt and find a new way of functioning.
- Alpha is activated by cold.
- Beta is activated by heat.

It is important to note that beta closes the cycle of para and alpha. One of the factors that play a role in illness is the inability of beta to install itself in the normal chronological cycle of the ANS.

Figure 3 shows the normal cycle of the ANS. Serotonin is the autacoid of para and histamine the autacoid of alpha. Autacoids are chemical substances that act as hormones and cause-specific physiological changes.[14]

Figure 4 shows the normal cycle of the ANS represented by the broken line. The solid line depicts a scenario, where there is a dysfunction in the normal cycle of the ANS. Para is initially at the same level, but due to a rise in histamine there is an increase in and a prolonged activity of alpha. As there is a rise in alpha, there is an increase in beta activity also. Due to this disturbance, the normal level of para has increased.

As described in *The Theory of Endobiogeny*, Volume 1, page 37.

(© *2014 Systems Biology Research Group based on the work of SIMEPI, based on the work of SFEM*, based on the concepts of Dr Christian Duraffourd)

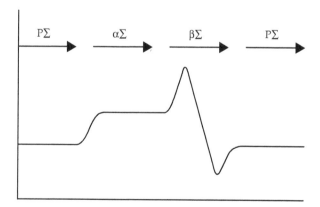

Figure 3. Normal cycle of the ANS.

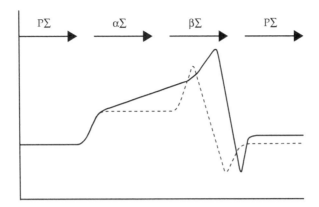

Figure 4. Dysfunction in the cycle of the ANS.

Important betasympathetic effects, signs and symptoms

- Centrally, beta increases alertness and mental activity, anxiety, panic attacks and obsessive behaviour due to high TRH (central beta).
- Discharge/release of stress peripherally; sometimes in an abrupt manner, e.g. vomiting, bowel evacuation, urination. Beta is the release mechanism.
- Warm hands.
- If beta is elevated, it may cause palpitations.
- Beta is a catabolic system, so it can be linked to weight loss.

The way para, alpha and beta work together

In relation to the sphincter of Oddi regulation

As with all other sphincters, the functional regulation of the sphincter of Oddi depends on the coordination of the three divisions of the autonomic nervous system para, alpha and beta.

Parasympathetic

The parasympathetic system sets the basal tone (resting tone) of the sphincter.

Alphasympathetic

As seen in Figure 3, alphasympathetic follows parasympathetic activity in the sequence. Alpha follows para and regulates its action in an obligatory sequence.

Alpha

- Overrides the parasympathetic activity.
- Raises the basal tone of the sphincter.
- Determines the closing tone of the sphincter and also its duration of closure.[13]

As discussed previously, the alphasympathetic system is a constrictive system. In relation to the sphincters of the digestive system, alpha is responsible for the closing tone of the sphincters. Therefore, if alpha is high, it will cause the sphincters to constrict, impairing the flow of secretions of the organs such as bile and pancreatic juices, thus, resulting in impaired digestive function. Alpha also reduces intestinal motility and in so doing playing a role in constipation.

The betasympathetic

This is the release mechanism. Beta very briefly increases the tension induced by alpha until its autolysis, which, like an explosion, releases the tension, allowing the sphincter to open releasing the secretions: bile and pancreatic juices.[13]

From what we have discussed so far, it is evident that stressors (aggressors) will cause alterations at the level of the autonomic nervous system and also as we will shortly see, at the level of the endocrine system.

Stress affects the whole system

Psychoneuroimmunology (PNI) research has demonstrated that there is a link between increased central activity (psychological stress perception) and downstream endocrine and immune changes.[15] Whether the stress is acute or chronic is significant. Short term acute stress is far less damaging and the organism is able to adapt. As we will see in the section on the endocrine system, chronic stress is far more damaging and causes pronounced endocrinometabolic changes that effect the tissues and cells of the body, causing and exacerbating inflammation. This is an important part of the puzzle in terms of IBD.

Stress also affects the foetus

Stress has a major impact on the developing foetus and there is a link between the stress that the mother is subjected to in pregnancy and postnatal disease.[15] Research describes maternal stress as a possible perinatal programming agent.

> Perinatal programming occurs when characteristics of the in-utero environment, independent of genetic susceptibility, influence foetal development to permanently organize or imprint physiological systems.[16]

It is believed that intrauterine stress hormones rise with prenatal maternal stress and that the effect of these stress hormones is to alter the natural immunoregulatory mechanisms and in so doing cause an increased risk in developing inflammatory diseases.[16]

Histamine: the autacoid of alpha

Histamine is an excitatory neuro-transmitter which is made from the amino acid histidine.[17] As an excitatory neurotransmitter, histamine promotes wakefulness by stimulating the basal forebrain, thus interfering with the normal sleep cycle.[18] Patients with elevated histamine levels can often complain that they still feel tired after sleeping.

The histamine/stress connection

Stress increases histamine. It has been shown that mast cells are activated by stressors.[19] These stressors can either be emotional, physical or environmental. Once activated, they release an array of over 50 potent molecules, including histamine, which cause or further aggravate inflammation.[20] In fact, histamine is a major mediator of inflammation and plays a key role in inflammatory diseases like IBD. In relation to the colon, specifically, acute stress has been found to increase histamine levels of mast cells in the colon, resulting in functional disturbances.[19]

Histamine is important

Histamine is not just a major mediator of inflammation. As with all things, it is a question of balance. It is all relative. Histamine has three important roles:

1. congestion
2. repair
3. defence

The body defends itself emotionally and physically through the action of histamine. Histamine plays an essential immune role helping to regulate the immune response. It does this via its effects on macrophages, dendritic cells, T Lymphocytes, B lymphocytes and endothelial cells, which are all effected by and also secrete histamine.[21] Histamine has the ability to effect immunity in different ways depending on the type of receptor-activated, ultimately having an effect on a specialised subsets of T helper cells (TH1 and TH2). Therefore, histamine effects both innate and adaptive immune cells.[22]

The effect that histamine has centrally (in the brain) is interesting to say the least. Histamine releasing neurons of the brain are located exclusively in the tuberomammillary nucleus of the posterior hypothalamus, where they project to practically all brain regions. Histamine has many functions at brain level. It plays a particular role in the control of excitability and plasticity. In addition to this, histamine has a close relationship with other neurotransmitter systems in the brain, which through a complex network regulate sleep-wake cycles, circadian and feeding rhythms, immunity, learning and memory.[23]

The alpha, histamine, beta and cortisol connection

This connection, if understood well, will enable you to treat your patients at a much deeper level. What is histamines role in all of this? Let's break this down and then connect all the dots. As seen in Figure 5, alpha stimulates histamine release and histamine prolongs the action of alpha and at the same time retards beta. In this situation there is not enough cortisol to block the histamine, so a positive feedback cycle occurs and a vicious stress-induced histamine cycle is put into motion. In order to obtain the best results from treatment, you will need to address each pathway. You will need to choose specific plants or supplements that can reduce alpha, reduce histamine and support the adrenals.

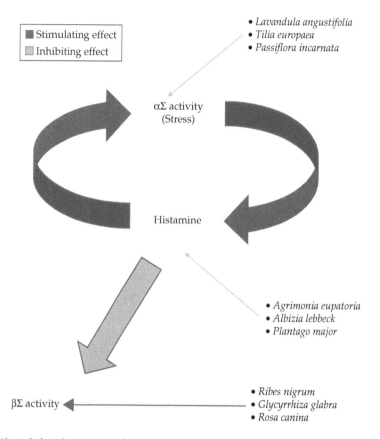

Figure 5. The alpha, histamine, beta and cortisol connection.

Serotonin: the autacoid of para

Serotonin is well known for its effects on emotional states. However, there is more, much more, to this interesting neurotransmitter. In endobiogenic medicine, serotonin is central para. When we look at the functional biology indexes, we will discuss the peripheral serotonin index and you will see that if serotonin is high peripherally it is low centrally and vice versa. As the autacoid of para, serotonin prolongs the action of the parasympathetic nervous system and will consequently be all the more present when a high para precedes the illness.[24]

CHAPTER THREE

Plant medicines that act on the autonomic nervous system

Table 2. Alphasympatholytic plants[25,26,27]

Plant	Form used	Other actions
Lavandula angustifolia	Essential oil, tincture, fluid extract, infusion	known as the 'super alpha-blocker': alphasympatholytic and mildly parasympatholytic, antiseptic against strep and staph (respiratory, intestinal, biliary, genitourinary, and cutaneous), choleretic and diuretic. Relaxes sphincter of Oddi.
Melissa officinalis	Essential oil, tincture, fluid extract, infusion	alphasympatholytic, digestive, antispasmodic, choleretic, anxiolytic (prolongs GABA activity), neuro-calmative, cognitive enhancer (muscarinic and nicotinic receptors), enhances attention and memory, inhibits TSH. Relaxes sphincter of Oddi.
Passiflora incarnata	Tincture, fluid extract, infusion	alphasympatholytic, musculotropic and neurotropic antispasmodic (digestive and cardiovascular), sedative without somnolence or reduction of vigilance, GABA-ergic, anti-epileptic.

Table 3. Parasympatholytic plants[25,27,28]

Plant	Form used	Other actions
Thymus vulgaris	Essential oil, tincture, infusion	powerful parasympatholytic, adrenal stimulant (essential oil form only) anti-inflammatory, antibacterial, anti-fungal, antiviral, diuretic and choleretic.
Artemisia dracunculus	Essential oil	antispasmodic, vagolitic, parasympatholytic, antihistamine, anti-inflammatory, pelvic decongestant, splanchnic decongestant, antibacterial and antiviral (ENT, digestive, genitourinary tropisms).
Chamomilla recutita	Essential oil, tincture, infusion	parasympatholytic, vagolytic, alphasympatholytic, choleretic, antacid, digestive antispasmodic, antihistamine, antibacterial, anti-fungal, anti-parasitic, sedative, antispasmodic, anti-inflammatory, decongestant: hepatic, splanchnic, pelvic.
Achillea millefolium	Essential oil, tincture, infusion	parasympatholytic, vagolytic, digestive antispasmodic, carminative, antigastritic, choleretic, hepatoprotector, a pelvic decongestant (venous stimulation), anti-inflammatory, pelvic antispasmodic, progesterone-like *without inhibiting LH*, aldosterone antagonist, hemostatic, anti-haemorrhagic, inhibits platelet aggregation, antithrombotic, anti-haemorrhagic, anti-inflammatory, antiseptic, hemostatic, astringent;

Table 4. Beta-mimetic plants[25,27,29]

Plant	Form used	Other actions
Ribes nigrum GM	Glycerine macerate D1 dilution	glucocorticoid stimulant (adrenal cortex), anti-allergic, anti-inflammatory.
Rosa canina GM	Glycerine macerate D1 dilution	Adrenal cortex stimulant, betasympathomimetic, anti-infectious for ENT.
Glycyrrhiza glabra	Tincture, fluid extract, decoction	Anti-inflammatory (digestive, respiratory), anti-allergic (respiratory), expectorant, digestive antispasmodic, decongestant, antacid, anti-gastritic, oestrogenic, aldosterone-like (favours sodium retention), potentiates effects of corticosteroids.

Table 5. Antihistamine plants[25,30]

Plant	Form used	Other actions
Artemisia dracunculus	Essential oil	antihistamine, anti-inflammatory, antioxidant, digestive antispasmodic, vagolytic, antiemetic, aperitif, carminative, splanchnic decongestant, pelvic decongestant, Antibacterial and Antiviral.
Albizzia lebbeck	Tincture	Antihistamine, found to have a protective effect against histamine-induced bronchospasm. Protects the adrenal glands against the negative effects of histamine.
Plantago major	Tincture, infusion	Anti-allergic, digestive anti-inflammatory. Anti-tussive, mucolytic, expectorant, antispasmodic, antigastritic, antacid, astringent, digestive antispasmodic, anti-ulcer: gastric and duodenal.

CHAPTER FOUR

Case studies related to the autonomic nervous system: workbook exercises

*S*elect the symptoms that are linked to parasympathetic, alphasympathetic and betasympathetic imbalances.

Case 1

A 22-year-old patient, male, presenting with post-prandial somnolence, which can occur after any meal, finds it hard to pass urine and it can take 2 to 3 minutes before urine starts to flow. There is also pain when passing urine. The pain can last until he finishes passing urine, or it can be present just at the beginning. When the urine comes, it comes with force.

The patient also suffers from difficulty in opening his bowels. He opens his bowels one to three times daily, but they can take up to 15 minutes to open. There is incomplete bowel evacuation even when he does open his bowels.

Case 2

A 23-year-old patient, female, presenting with digestive problems, sleep disturbance and fatigue. GI symptoms include cramping, severe bloating and nausea in the evening. Symptoms started 10 years ago after a parasitic infection contracted from her cat; she was 15 years old at the time. The patient does not remember exactly what parasite. Intolerance tests at Royal Free Hospital showed intolerance to gluten and dairy. She opens bowels four times a week only. When she opens her bowels, she does completely empty them. Suffers from lots of odourless flatulence. Every Saturday morning as soon as rises she has diarrhoea. Also, headaches on weekends. Takes two paracetamols every weekend. Work schedule: 8.30 am to 7.30 pm but usually stays until 8.30 or 9 pm.

Cases explained

Case 1

High para

- Post-prandial somnolence is related to an excess of para. Para is stimulated by eating, so this will reinforce the parasympathetic activity, which is already high in this patient.

High alpha and delayed and insufficient beta

- Finds it hard to pass urine and can take 2 or 3 minutes before the urine starts to flow. Alpha is a constrictive system causing contraction of the internal urethral sphincter; thus, the urine will not flow freely. The delayed and deficient beta state is responsible for maintaining the high alpha, and the sphincter will not relax in order to allow the urine to flow. Once beta, which is delayed, is activated sufficiently, then the urine starts to flow.
- The pain when passing urine is related to the constrictive effects of alpha, i.e. the inability of the urine to flow freely. Once beta is adequately activated and the urine flows freely the pain diminishes. This is why the pain can last for the duration of urination or simply be present at the beginning. It depends on when in the duration of urination beta will be adequately activated.
- When the urine comes, it comes with force. This is related to beta. Beta is the release mechanism. Once activated sufficiently, the urine will flow with force. The greater the force, the greater the beta activity is. So, in this case beta is retarded, as it is not installing itself in the normal chronological cycle of events.
- The difficulty in opening the bowels is most likely related to high alpha, as alpha reduces intestinal motility. There is an incomplete evacuation of the bowels as there is a dysfunction in the rhythm of para, alpha and beta thus disrupting peristalsis.

Case 2

The parasitic infection is an aggressor. It is a factor that modified the terrain. A trigger. There may have been other imbalances in the terrain that made the patient more susceptible to reacting in this way to the parasite, but the parasite was a significant aggressor. When taking a thorough case history, in such a patient, it is important to look at the history before the parasitic infection occurred. This will provide clues, as to the imbalances in terrain that were pre-existing. The fact that the patient was 15 years old at the time is significant, as puberty is a sensitive time when the organism is changing and thus more vulnerable.

High para

- Nausea is related to a high para-state. In this case, the nausea is present in the evening, and this is not a coincidence, it is because the parasympathetic system is higher in the evening and at night time. Para rises at night to prepare the body for sleep.

High alpha and low beta

- Opens bowels four times a week only. Alpha reduces intestinal motility. It is a constrictive system and constricts the sphincter of Oddi, thus interfering with the flow of bile and pancreatic juices.

Beta discharge

- Every Saturday morning as soon as she rises, she has diarrhoea. Also, headaches on the weekends. This occurs because it is the weekend and the patient relaxes; she is able to let go. As a result, there is a sufficient and pronounced beta discharge which results in diarrhoea and headache. Remember that the beta system is the release mechanism. The headache occurs because there is a dilation of the blood vessels induced by beta, and as a result, an abrupt increase in blood flow to the head. The high alpha was constricting the blood vessels all week and impeding circulation.

CHAPTER FIVE

Drainage

What is drainage?

Drainage is the process of sustaining or stimulating the secretory or excretory functions of our different eliminatory or emunctory organs which are the

- Hepatobiliary apparatus
- Digestive tract
- Pancreas
- Kidneys
- Skin
- Respiratory tract

For the purpose of this book, we will be focusing specifically on the drainage of the hepatobiliary apparatus, digestive tract and pancreas.

What is the purpose of drainage?

The purpose of drainage is to improve the function of or detoxification of an eliminatory or emunctory organ.

An emunctory organ is an organ that rids the body of waste. An example is the colon. If the colon is not draining properly, and the patient becomes congested, this will lead to toxicity. The organism will not be able to detoxify appropriately and will reabsorb toxins back into the system.

How to drain an organ!

Therapeutic drainage involves stimulating an emunctory organ to detoxify by increasing either:

- the quantity of its secretion, or
- the concentration
  - of all of its components, or
  - of only one or several of these[31]

Drainage occurs physiologically in the organism, either as a regular, continuous basic activity or as a stimulated activity with variable intensity depending on adaptation or adaptability demands.[31]

Examples of physiological drainage

1. The acceleration of natural elimination, which can occur in a sudden, one-off episode of diarrhoea.
2. The externalisation of normally hidden secretions, such as rhinorrhoea or unusual outbreaks of seborrhoea due to emotional causes.
3. The occurrence of internal cleansing—phagocytosis.

Role of medicinal plants in drainage

There are many plants with varying effects, that can improve the drainage of the emunctory organs implicated either directly or indirectly in the condition in question. These medicinal plants can be categorised as

- **Choleretics:** agents that stimulate bile production by the hepatocytes in the liver.[27]
- **Cholagogues:** agents that stimulate the release of bile that has already been formed in the biliary system. Therefore, increase biliary evacuation.[27]
- **Plants with mixed activity:** (choleretic and cholagogue).
- **Antispasmodics:** these plants have specific effects ANS imbalances. For example, on the sphincter of Oddi addressing the spasm that can occur.

Drainage is more of a superficial treatment

It is important to discover what the true mechanism of the congestion is by looking at the underlying factors involved. However, drainage, is very useful and effective if done properly. It is a useful treatment modality.

The levels of treatment are as follows

1. Symptomatic treatment, e.g. prescribing an anti-inflammatory or antibacterial agent

2. Drainage
3. Addressing imbalances at the level of the autonomic nervous system
4. Addressing imbalances at the level of the endocrine system

Drainage is one of the therapeutic axes, and when it is performed properly, it complements the etiological treatment, which is designed to correct the underlying mechanisms of the disease linked to the pre-critical terrain.

Drainage is adjustable

- in intensity
- in selectivity

Drainage can be varied in intensity with plant medicines; you can choose to simply regulate and maintain a function, correct and support a function or, in a more intense form, force the function of a particular emunctory or group of emunctories.

Drainage can be adjusted in selectivity. You can choose to

1. Drain an emunctory organ
This involves stimulating the organ directly involved in the condition in question. This is a specific symptomatic action which is directed, either at the organ's own function or at the relationship between the organ in question and another organ. This is referred to as assisting the function of or supporting organ.[31]

2. Drain the *organism*
This involves the drainage of several emunctories, and targets one or several functions. It is part of the aetiological treatment of the disease. This type of drainage will aid in the regulation of various organs that are implicated in the metabolic imbalance concerned.[31]

In metabolic pathology, the main organs affected are

- The digestive tract
- The hepatobiliary system
- The pancreas[31]

And to a lesser extent

- The respiratory system
- The renal system
- The skin[31]

When to drain?

In some instances, it would not be wise to carry out drainage. Drainage should not be performed routinely without careful thought and planning for the following reasons:

a. Any choleretic prescription will increase liver detoxification. As a result, it will accelerate the catabolism of the steroid and thyroid hormones which can be enough to induce a lack of hormonal efficiency in relation to the demands of the organism.
b. **It is important to note:** liver congestion is always in response to a metabolic need for hyperactivity. 'Congestion is an adaptive physiological phenomenon aimed at increasing the activity and output of a tissue, an organ or a group of organs'. It allows a tissue to be over-nourished or to have its nourishment prolonged. Therefore, do not automatically drain the liver because it is congested.[31]

Drainage of the emunctories

Emunctory drainage can be implemented when there is a nonspecific overload on the organism, or if the organic functions are not known. It is also indicated in patients who are spasmophiliac, have no specific imbalance or suffer from generally sluggish elimination. In these cases, it is advisable to perform a general drainage of the emunctories, focused on the problem identified.

Drainage of the organism

Should only be performed when there is a certainty of the diagnosis and indeed, the mechanism of the condition present. There must be a good understanding of the organs of detoxification that are involved in the metabolic imbalance, and the practitioner must be able to identify the main organ implicated in the illness.

Drainage of the organ

It is important to emphasise that one must never force the activity of an organ that seems deficient. It is essential to identify the cause and purpose of the deficiency, as the deficiency may be part of a defence system that the organism has put into place to protect itself.

Congestion related to autonomic nervous dysregulation

As discussed in detail in the previous chapters, dysregulation in the autonomic nervous system causes dysfunction in the organism. The dysfunction at the level of the autonomic nervous system is implicated in the phenomenon of congestion. We have already discussed this when we spoke about the sphincter of Oddi. If there is a high alpha, there is a constriction in the organism and a constriction of the sphincters. When this is present, a patient can present with a significant splanchnic congestion. We will look at specific examination techniques later on, showing how you can examine patients in order to determine whether or not splanchnic congestion is present.

In order to address drainage in such patients, we need to consider the imbalances that exist at the level of the autonomic nervous system. If you simply drain the organs, e.g. liver and gallbladder, using cholagogues you may not obtain the best results. You need to consider reducing alphasympathetic activity as it may be the driving factor. You may also wish to stimulate betasympathetic activity in order to release the congestion.

The fascinating thing about plant medicines is that we have so many to choose from. Each plant having multiple actions. It is possible to select a plant that can drain the splanchnic region and at the same time have a beta-mimetic effect. *Menyanthes trifoliata* is such a plant.

Alternatively, you may wish to use *Ribes nigrum* gemmotherapy D1 as it is a truly fantastic plant for sustaining beta activity and supporting the adrenal cortex. In addition, you could use *Lavandula angustifolia* or *Melissa officinalis* to relax the sphincter of Oddi and to reduce alphasympathetic activity.

These are just some examples of plants that you may choose. Externally you may wish to give a preparation containing essential oils that the patient can use to massage the splanchnic area or abdominal region with. Such a formula will depend on the aim of your treatment. If you are dealing with a patient who has recurrent bowel spasm you may wish to use essential oils such as:

- *Lavandula angustifolia* EO
- *Levisticum officinale* EO
- *Thymus vulgaris* EO
- *Chamomila recutita* EO

Remember, over time, if using essential oils on the skin, they will absorb into the body and have a systemic effect.

Drainage of the Intestines, pancreas and hepatobiliary system

Intestinal drainage

Intestinal drainage can play a role along the whole length of the digestive tract.

This can be achieved by

- Increasing transit time which is relevant in cases of impaired elimination
- Or by slowing down transit
- Or by improving the quality of absorption

Intestinal physiology

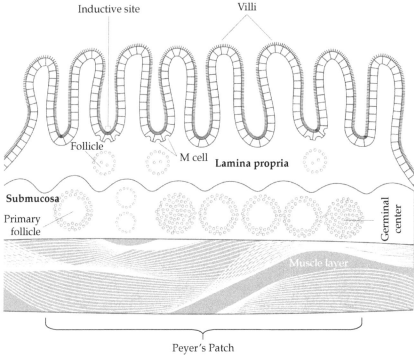

Figure 6. Structural components of the mucosal barrier.

Plant medicines used to drain the intestines[25]

- *Vaccinium myrtillus* (bilberry).
- *Malva sylvestris* (blue mallow).
- *Juglans regia* (green walnut leaf).
- *Cinnamomum zeylanicum* (cinnamon).
- *Rumex crispus* (yellow dock).
- Illite clay (green clay)—this has phenomenal detoxifying and healing properties. We will discuss the use of green clay in detail later on in this book.

Pancreatic drainage

Pancreatic drainage

It is important to remember that the pancreas has both endocrine and exocrine functions. It plays two distinct metabolic roles related to:

a. Insulin
b. Protein, lipid and carbohydrate metabolism

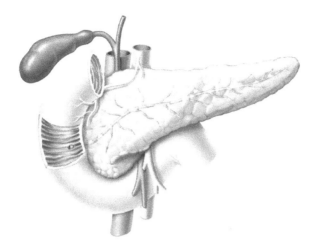

Figure 7. Pancreatic physiology.

Treatment

Plant medicines that act on the pancreas can either act on the endocrine or exocrine pancreas or have a mixed effect acting on both the endocrine and exocrine pancreas.

Plants affecting the exocrine pancreas

- *Rubus fructicosus* (blackberry): hypoglycaemiant,[32,33] indirect anti-diabetic, pancreatic drainer.[25]
- *Fumaria officinalis* (fumitory): pancreatic drainer.[25]
- *Trigonella foenum-graecum* (fenugreek): hypoglycaemiant, anti-diabetic, hyperinsulinemic, stimulates the endocrine pancreas.[34]

Plants affecting the endocrine pancreas

Plants reduce insulin resistance

- *Agrimonia eupatoria* (agrimony)
- *Juglans regia* (green walnut)

Plants which reduce insulin

- *Malva sylvestris* (blue mallow): more effective if used after meals.

Plants with mixed action, affecting both endocrine and exocrine pancreas

- *Cichorium intybus* (chicory)
- *Nasturtium officinale* (watercress)

- *Olea europaes* (olive leaf)
- *Eucalyptus globules* (eucalyptus)
- *Juglans regia* (green walnut)
- *Agrimonia eupatoria*

Liver

Liver drainage

The livers importance in metabolism is immense. Indeed, it is located at the cross-roads of metabolism as a whole, being involved in anabolic and catabolic functions of the organism. The liver also plays a vital role in detoxifying the organism.

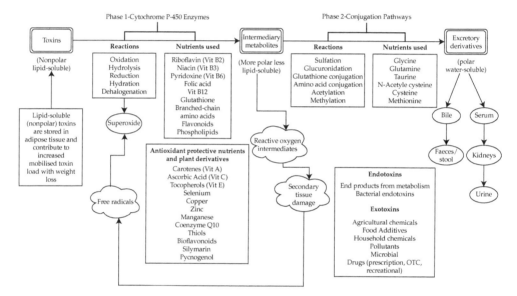

Figure 8. Detoxification pathways.

Plants that drain the liver:

- *Cynare scolymus* (artichoke)
- *Arcticum lappa* (burdock)
- *Fumaria officinale* (fumitory)
- *Raphanus niger* (black radish)
- *Rosmarinus officinalis* (rosemary)
- *Carduus marianus* (milk thistle)

CHAPTER SIX

Exocrine pancreatic insufficiency: symptomatology

Definition

Exocrine pancreatic insufficiency (EPI) occurs when there is inadequate pancreatic enzyme activity. This can occur due to the following reasons:

1. insuffcient enzyme production
2. insuffcient enzyme activation
3. early enzyme degradation

EPI can be classified as primary or secondary:

- In primary EPI there is either a lack of exocrine pancreatic tissue or an insufficient innervation of the exocrine pancreas.
- In secondary EPI, there is sufficient production and release of pancreatic enzymes, but the enzymes are not fully active. This can occur, either due to anatomical changes related to surgery, or due to inappropriate activation or inactivation of these enzymes.[35]

Enzymes produced in the pancreas

- Pancreatic protease (trypsin and chymotrypsin). These are proteolytic enzymes.
- Pancreatic amylase. Required for the digestion of carbohydrates.
- Pancreatic lipase. Required for the digestion of fats.

Digestion of lipids

The digestion of lipids is almost totally dependent on pancreatic lipase; therefore, if there is an insufficiency of lipase, there will be fat intolerance. Indeed, the first signs of exocrine pancreatic insufficiency are those related to lipase insufficiency.

The following signs and symptoms may be present depending on the severity of the lipase deficiency: sticky stools, unformed, pasty, runny like mud, floating stools, fatty stools (steatorrhoea) with an acceleration of transit and diarrhoea due to the lubricating effect of the undigested fats. Following this, weight loss and malabsorption of fat-soluble vitamins (A, D, E and K) can occur. B12 deficiency is also common, resulting in microcytic anaemia and osteomalacia.[36]

Digestion of carbohydrates

Amylase is the main pancreatic glycolytic enzyme. When pancreatic amylase is insufficient, the parotid glands will increase their secretion of alpha-amylase in order to compensate. Parasympathetic activity will also rise as para innervates the parotids and controls their secretion. As a result of this, initially there will be greater parotid activity, hence an increase in salivary secretions and later on if the imbalance persists and is not rectified this will result in hypertrophy of the parotids which is the result of major vagal reactivity. Inappropriate digestion of carbohydrates leads to excessive fermentation in the digestive tract resulting in pain and flatulence.

Digestion of proteins

Insufficiency of proteolytic enzymes is rarer and more episodic. When this occurs, there is putrefaction of proteins in the intestine resulting in foul-smelling flatulence.

Vagal stimulation

Exocrine pancreatic insufficiency leads to vagal overstimulation, effecting not only the parotids, but the whole organism, resulting in

- recurring ENT and respiratory infections as a result of disturbances in the formation of intestinal plasma cells, which migrate through the lymphatic system and produce secretory IgA.
- recurring hiccups due to the irritation of the diaphragm caused by the vagal overstimulation.
- episodes of urticaria caused by poor functioning of the emunctories (usually the liver and exocrine pancreas).
- post-prandial somnolence due to the high para-state.
- generalised sweating after meals, early at night and around 5 am. Remember that para rises at night and also remember that the act of eating will stimulate para

even more. This is generally the case with high para and not specific to exocrine pancreatic insufficiency.

- imbalance of the microbiome of the bowels.
- recurring fungal infections of the digestive tract, especially the anus, genital area, palms and soles of the feet.
- craving for sugar, as there can be reactive hyperinsulinism.

The exocrine pancreatic insufficiency causes a drop in the energy of the organism. The resultant effect is an overstimulation of the thyroid in order to rectify the lack of energy, and thus an appeal to insulin is made leading to secondary hyperinsulinism.[36] This hyperinsulinism has negative consequences, as insulin increases inflammation.

Signs on clinical examination

- There will be swelling of the orifice of the parotid ducts. Upon examination, sialorrhoea will be present, completely filling the oral cavity.
- Upon palpation and if severe, by observation of an increased volume of parotid glands.
- Tonsillar signs.
- Loss of the lingual papillae and fissures present on the tongue.
- White coating of the posterior tongue implies dysbiosis of the colon.
- White coating of anterior tongue implies dysbiosis of the small intestine.
- Signs of intestinal disturbance; the pancreas plays a vital role in digestion; thus, it plays a significant role in the provision of nutrients to the intestines. As discussed above, if the food is not digested appropriately dysbiosis can develop. In addition to this, the pancreas plays an important role in the inflammatory process due to the reactive hyperinsulinism that can occur.
- Signs of splanchnic congestion. Congestion of liver, gallbladder and pancreas. Please see Chapter 16 on endobiogenic examination.
- There may be pain on palpation of the pancreas.

We must not forget the importance of the autonomic nervous system imbalances involved in the dysregulation of the pancreas and the involvement of the sphincter of Oddi as discussed in detail previously.

Phytotherapy treatment

When prescribing plant medicines in the treatment of exocrine pancreatic insufficiency, the practitioner must keep in mind three fundamental points:

1. If the sphincter of Oddi is involved, which is almost always the case, it is essential to prescribe antispasmodic plants and at the same time, drain the liver and the gall bladder.

3. If the signs of pancreatic insufficiency are mild or are linked to overeating, you can stimulate pancreatic secretion as well as liver and gall bladder activity with parasympathomimetic plants: e.g. *Fumaria officinalis*, *Rosmarinus officinalis* and *Mentha piperita*.

4. If the symptomatology is very clear, pancreatic secretion must not be stimulated, as the pancreas may become exhausted and thus aggravate the patient's state. Congestive states resulting from conflict of para and alpha can be treated by plants that are vagolytic and alphasympatholytic: e.g. *Lavandula angustifolia* and *Anthemis nobilis*.[36]

Treatment strategies and plants used

Table 6. Hepatopancreatic drainage[25,36]

Plant	Form used	Action
Fumaria officinalis	Infusion, tincture, fluid extract	Choleretic, supports the exocrine pancreas
Agrimonia eupatoria	Infusion, tincture, fluid extract	Astringent, supports the exocrine and endocrine pancreas
Arctium lappa	Decoction, tincture, fluid extract	Choleretic, supports the exocrine and endocrine pancreas

Table 7. Correction of autonomic nervous system imbalance. Specifically in relation to spasm of the sphincter of Oddi[25,36]

Plant	Form used	Action
Lavandula angustifolia	Tincture, fluid extract, essential oil, infusion	Vagolytic and sympatholytic
Anthemis nobilis	Tincture, fluid extract, essential oil, infusion	Vagolytic and sympatholytic
Angelica archangelica	Tincture, fluid extract, Essential oil, decoction	Vagolytic and sympatholytic
Ocimum basilicum	Tincture, fluid extract, essential oil, infusion	Vagolytic and sympatholytic

Table 8. Vagolytic[25,36]

Plant	Form used	Action
Thymus vulgaris	Infusion, tincture, fluid extract, essential oil	Vagolytic
Artemisia dracunculus	Essential oil	Vagolytic
Cuminum cyminum	Essential oil	Vagolytic
Carum carvi	Essential oil	Vagolytic

Table 9. Symptomatic treatment[25,36]

Plant	Form used	Action
Vaccinium myrtillus fr	Tincture, fluid extract	Anti-inflammatory, astringent, antiseptic
Juglans regia fol	Decoction, tincture, fluid extract	Anti-inflammatory, astringent, antiseptic
Cinnamomum zeylanicum	Essential oil	Intestinal antiseptics
Eugenia caryophyllata	Decoction, tincture, fluid extract, essential oil	Intestinal antiseptics

The following adjuvant treatments are very helpful:

• Enzyme substitution: this includes the use of digestive and systemic enzymes. These two types of enzyme preparations work differently. A digestive enzyme should be taken at the start of a meal. These enzymes assist in the digestion of various foods depending on the type of enzymes prescribed. Most digestive enzymes are broad-spectrum enzymes. These supplements can support the pancreas and indirectly have an effect on reducing parasympathetic activity by reducing the overactivity of para, which has been induced by an initial lack of exocrine pancreatic activity. Systemic enzymes should be taken approximately 1 hour before a meal usually two or three times daily. The stomach should be empty when taking these enzymes, as the aim is for the enzymes to be absorbed into the system and have a systemic effect. If they are taken with a meal, they will simply be used up in the digestion of that food.
• Restoration of intestinal flora using probiotics and specific diet protocols, which we will discuss later on.
• Counter fermentation using therapeutic agents like charcoal and green clay. We will look specifically at the highly beneficial medicinal actions of green clay later on.

Systemic enzymes

In my practice I have found that systemic enzyme preparations have an important place in the treatment of several conditions. Specifically, in relation to digestive disorders, systemic enzymes play a key role in the treatment of the following: exocrine pancreatic insufficiency, bloating, floating stools, inflammation (particularly enteropathic arthritis) seen in Crohn's and ulcerative colitis, scar tissue due to chronic ulceration of the bowel and abdominal adhesions related to abdominal surgery. Systemic enzymes can play a key therapeutic role in many other conditions which are outside the scope of this book.

There are many different types of systemic enzymes, and there can be an overlap with digestive enzymes depending on how they are used as mentioned above. We will touch upon a few of these now in order to give you an idea of how they can benefit patients. In my practice I often use specific systemic enzyme formulas which contain a blend of several enzymes.

Bromelain, serrapeptase, trypsin and chymotrypsin

Bromelain has been used as a safe phytotherapeutic agent in folk medicine for many years. Bromelain has been shown to have marked anti-inflammatory and immuno-modulatory properties. It also has antithrombotic and fibrinolytic effects, as well as enhancing circulation and improving wound healing.[37]

Serrapeptase has earnt the name 'the miracle enzyme' as patients have found this enzyme beneficial for a whole host of inflammatory issues as well as conditions where there is excessive mucus build-up and congestion. In relation to trismus caused by surgical removal of impacted molars; a review of five studies demonstrate that ser-rapeptase was more successful than corticosteroids in improving this condition.[38] A further study looking at trypsin chymotrypsin and serratiopeptidase demonstrated that these three enzymes exhibit pronounced anti-inflammatory effects. In addition to this, these enzymes actually reduced the ulcer index significantly as compared to aspirin which has the tendency to increase ulcer index. The study states that the anti-inflammatory activity of all of these enzymes were dose dependent.[39]

A trypsin and chymotrypsin combination is a widely used systemic enzyme for-mula taken to assist in the recovery and repair of traumatic injuries as well as surgical trauma. Research shows that this combination is highly bioavailable while main-taining its therapeutic effects as an anti-inflammatory, anti-oedematous, fibrinolytic, antioxidant and anti-infective agent. In addition to this, it possesses analgesic proper-ties which makes it ideal in dealing with the pain associated with trauma recovery. Research shows that it is superior at promoting recovery and has greater anti-inflam-matory effect than several other enzyme formulas. Its efficacy and safety have been corroborated by substantial clinical trials.[40]

CHAPTER SEVEN

Introduction to the endocrine system

What is the endocrine system?

Classically, the endocrine system is seen to control the flow of information between different cells and tissue. The term 'endocrine' refers to the internal secretion of biologically active substances as appose to 'exocrine', which refers to secretion outside the body.

Endobiogenic medicine: the medicine of terrain

In endobiogenic medicine the endocrine system is seen to be the true manager, as it is the only system that manages itself and every other system in the organism. Only the endocrine system can provide all the necessary functions; indeed, the key to understanding the global metabolic functioning of the organism is to understand the intricate nature of the endocrine system and its effects on a cellular and tissular level. The endocrine system is deeper than the nervous system. It is the true architect. The autonomic nervous system helps regulate the endocrine system by regulating the intensity and duration of its function.

The action of the endocrine system is evident very early on in life. For example, its effect can be observed at the foetal stage of life. Indeed, the expression of the genetic potential of development and sexual differentiation is under the control of the various hormonal secretions.[41]

Hormonal mechanisms also play an important role in

- all phases of morphological transformation of the individual
  - puberty
  - menopause and male menopause (andropause)
  - growth
  - pregnancy
- in all behavioural disorders associated with endocrine disease
- in all metabolic activity and its regulating mechanisms[41]

The responsibility of the endocrine system is vast and is evident through its mechanisms of operation and regulation. It plays an essential role in ensuring the functionality of the terrain. 'It alone totally responds to the rules that dictate the function of an organized system thanks to':[41]

- regulation of the vertical axes (feedback), including the intervention of the systems of adaptation
- regulation of the horizontal axes

The endocrine system assures a ceaseless liaison. Chronologically, sequentially, qualitatively and quantitatively between the whole and each part of the organism.
   It plays a constant role in

- the true aetiology of every disease
- the struggle against serious disease
- the cohabitation between the host and the disease[41]

The capital notion of threshold

This is a very important notion that must be understood and remembered within the endobiogenic model. Always remember this when evaluating the functional biology and treating patients.

What do we mean by threshold?

This is best explained with the use of examples.

Example 1: High threshold

When circulating oestrogen in the blood falls from say 50 to 48 pg/mL follicle-stimulating hormone (FSH) immediately rises. In this example, FSH is extremely responsive to the fall in oestrogen.

Example 2: Low threshold

In this case circulating oestrogen has to fall from 50 to 10 pg/mL in order to elicit the same response from FSH. Here, FSH is much slower to respond to the fall in oestrogen.

The capital notion of threshold can explain, for example, why some women develop fibroids very quickly and others very slowly. The formation of fibroids is not only dependant on oestrogen, but what is more important is the fact that the threshold has been modified in favour of FSH. FSH primes the cells, making them more receptive to oestrogen. Even though, in this example we are talking about fibroids and it may not seem relevant to digestive disorders; it is a good example which will help in the understanding of the concept of threshold. As we will see later on, FSH and oestrogen activity are linked to the autoimmune process seen in Crohn's disease.

The importance of relativity

Always think in relative terms.

- One hormone is relative to another
- One marker in functional biology is relative to another

Just because, e.g. testosterone appears to be low does not mean its action is small. Relative to oestrogen it may actually be high.

Central and peripheral

In endobiogenic medicine, we talk about central and peripheral activity. Central pertains to the brain and peripheral pertains to the body.

When we discussed the autonomic nervous system, we looked at the subdivisions para, alpha and beta, and we discussed the neurotransmitters. We mainly discussed peripheral activity.

Peripheral activity

- Parasympathetic—acetylcholine
- Alphasympathetic—noradrenalin
- Betasympathetic—adrenalin

Peripheral para is acetylcholine; peripheral alpha is noradrenaline; peripheral beta is adrenalin.

Central activity

- Parasympathetic—serotonin
- Alphasympathetic—dopamine
- Betasympathetic—TRH (thyrotropin-releasing hormone)

Central para is serotonin; central alpha is dopamine; central beta is TRH.

It is important to distinguish between the two (central and peripheral) when diagnosing and treating patients, as it is essential to target the pathways involved in order for the treatment to be successful.

The greater the central activity, the greater the demand for glucose is. This is because the more mental activity there is, the more fuel is needed to keep the brain active. Figure 9 shows the stimulatory effect that glucose has on the central activity. It is important to keep this in mind when we discuss the functional biology markers and examine the case histories later on.

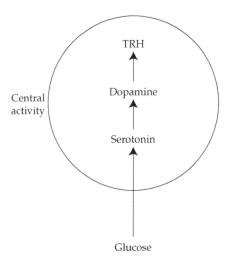

Figure 9. The effect of glucose on the central activity.

Endocrine axis and specific effects of hormones

In the next four chapters, we will look closely at the four endocrine vertical axes and the global effects of the hormones of the given axes. It is essential to understand the effects of each hormone outside its basic axis in order to fully appreciate the extent of the involvement of the endocrine system in the organism.

For the scope of this book, we will not be looking at all of the hormones in each axis but focus on the most pertinent relating to the digestive disorders discussed. There are two catabolic axes (corticotropic and thyrotropic) and two anabolic axes (gonadotropic and somatotropic).

CHAPTER EIGHT

Corticotropic axis

The corticotropic axis is a catabolic axis. It is the key initiator of the General Adaptation Syndrome, which is the physiological response of the body to aggression.

The corticotropic axis has a permissive influence upon the other endocrine axes. It does this through cortisol, which has a major metabolic role and has multiple actions on the organism. In endobiogenic medicine, the notion of permissivity is an important one, specifically in relation to cortisol. Cortisol can have two effects: either adaptive, where it can block the effects of other endocrine axes; or permissive, where it can facilitate and enhance the effects of other endocrine axes.[41] In terms of energy production, the corticotropic axis provides immediate energy.

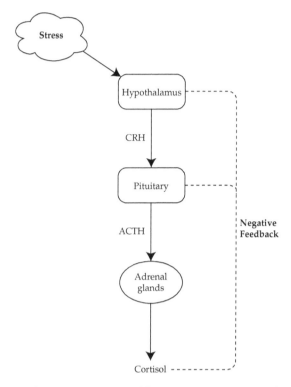

Figure 10. HPA axis. This axis is triggered by any aggression on the organism.
• CRH (cortocotropin-releasing hormone)
• ACTH (adrenocorticotropin hormone)
Negative feedback: cortisol inhibits both CRH and ACTH in order to regulate its own production.

ACTH

ACTH is secreted by the anterior pituitary gland and is secreted in response to any stressor, such as pain, fear, fever, hypoglycaemia etc. The circadian rhythm of ACTH is related to the light/dark cycle: the concentration of ACTH falls to its lowest between 11 pm and 2 am and increases until a morning peak between 6 am and 9 pm and from then on slowly declines.[42]

ACTH has the following actions:

• A major regulator of cortisol. Chronic stimulation of the adrenal cortex by ACTH leads to adrenocortical hyperplasia and hypertrophy.[43] whereas, ACTH deficiency results in decreased steroidogenesis and is accompanied by adrenocorticoid atrophy.[44]
• Can stimulate adrenal androgens and adrenal oestrogens.[43,45]

- ACTH enhances mobilisation of LDL cholesterol and stimulates the conversion of LDL cholesterol into various types of steroidogenic compounds.[46]
- Effects immunity: ACTH stimulates the production of T lymphocytes in the thymus gland.[47,48] ACTH has also been found to modulate the immune response by directly binding to receptors on leucocytes and enhancing a secondary (memory) cytotoxic response.[49] Overall ACTH appears to exhibit a regulatory effect on immunity: on one had it stimulates lymphocyte production and activity as described above and on the other hand reduces lymphocytes by its stimulation of cortisol which destroys them.[50]

ACTH receptors are located in terminal ileum, anus and breasts tissue. From an endobiogenic perspective, this is meaningful and can help explain the development of certain medical conditions. ACTH's participation in the disease process outside its vertical axes is significant, to say the least. We will look at this more closely soon.

Cortisol

Cortisol is a catabolic steroid hormone produced in the adrenal medulla. The circadian rhythm of cortisol is as follows: lowest at midnight and begins to rise between 2–3 am, peaking at about 8:30 am.[51]

Cortisol is essential for adaptation. Without it, the organism is not capable of adapting to aggression. As already mentioned, cortisol has two roles an adaptive role and a permissive role. The effects of cortisol on the organism are vast and complex. For the purposes of this book will only be discussing the effects related to the subject at hand.

Cortisol and immunity

Cortisol suppresses immunity: as mentioned in the section on ACTH, cortisol destroys lymphocytes. Research has demonstrated that a profound drop in lymphocytes and monocytes occurs with hydrocortisone administration.[52] Cortisol's effect on the destruction of lymphocytes is protective, against a dysregulation of the immune and inflammatory response.[50] Cortisol suppresses the immune response and inhibits natural killer cells.[53,54]

Indeed, a dysregulation of the HPA axis, which can occur at any level, has been linked to increased susceptibility to autoimmune disease and inflammation. The mechanism is related to low cortisol or glucocorticoid resistance caused by a diminished function in glucocorticoid receptors. In the case of the later, even if circulating cortisol levels are within the normal range or elevated there will still be an impaired function of cortisol at a tissular and cellular level, resulting in an impaired counter-regulation of the immune response.[55]

There are many factors to consider in the scenario of glucocorticoid resistance. Pathogens, chronic stress, chronic inflammation and chronic use of glucocorticoid medication, as well as genetic factors; more importantly, epigenetic factors, will affect the terrain of the organism.[55] Perinatal programming, in addition to behavioural programming, as a result of early-life experiences, can entrain a terrain which engenders a susceptibility to inflammatory and autoimmune disorders.

Several studies have now demonstrated that chronic stress and trauma play a major role in the relapse of inflammatory bowel disease (IBD). The nervous system effects the immune system of the organism, both systemically and locally at the gut mucosal level. The dysregulation of the HPA axis which we have already discussed, in conjunction with changes in the microbiome, mucosal mast cell activity and mediators such as corticotropin-releasing factor have been linked to the gastrointestinal inflammation seen in IBD.[56] Nicotinic, adrenergic and cholinergic receptor activity are all involved in this process. This suggests a complex interplay between the divisions of the autonomic nervous system: sympathetic and parasympathetic.[57]

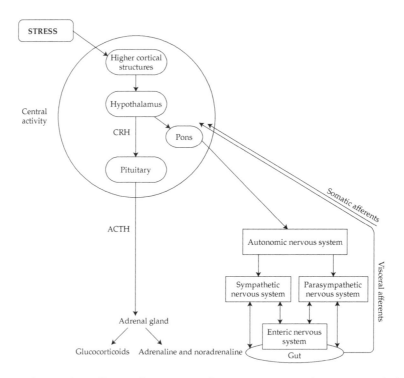

Figure 11. Shows the effects of stress on the gastrointestinal system and the pathways involved. ACTH—adrenocorticotrophic hormone; CRH—corticotrophin-releasing hormone.[56]

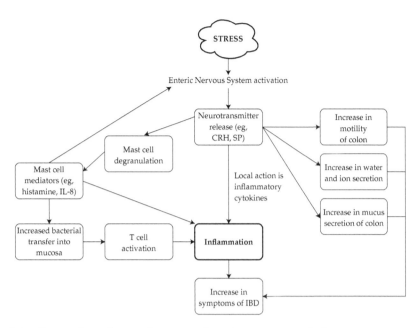

Figure 12. Shows the effects of stress-induced activation of the enteric nervous system on the gut in IBD. CRH—corticotrophin-releasing hormone; SP—substance P; IL—interleukin.[56]

These findings support the fact that psychological and environmental factors play an important role in the development of digestive disorders such as Crohn's and colitis. Indeed, Crohn's patients have a higher prevalence of psychiatric disorders.[57]

Effects on ANS

Cortisol has the ability to upregulate the number of betasympathetic receptors and in so doing amplifies the effects of adrenaline in adaptation.[50] It is also important to remember cortisol's antihistamine activity.

Effects on insulin and lipid storage

When cortisol is chronically elevated, it acts in a manner opposite to insulin by promoting insulin resistance.[58,59] Chronically elevated cortisol ultimately leads to an increase in lipid storage in specific regions of the body; face, trunk and interscapular region.[58]

Energy

Cortisol stimulates glycogenolysis and hepatic gluconeogenesis in order to raise much-needed blood glucose in times of stress. That, coupled with its anti-insulinic effect means that the glucose generated is denied entry to the non-vital organs and is instead reserved for the essential organs, e.g. heart and brain.

Thyroid

The permissive role of cortisol facilitates thyroid activity. However, when cortisol is chronically elevated and becomes maladaptive, it acts in a way that suppresses thyroid activity. It inhibits the conversion of T4 to active T3 and shunts T4 to reverse T3.[60] Ultimately cortisol inhibits function thyroid.

Effects on bone density

Cortisol exhibits profound effects on bone metabolism. It reduces bone density by increasing osteoclast activity, which in turn leads to an increase in bone resorption.[61,62] Furthermore, cortisol inhibits bone formation by reducing osteoblast activity.[62]

Surgery increases cortisol levels

It is important to note that cortisol levels rise substantially as a result of surgical procedures. This is important to consider when treating patients who undergo surgery, in order to formulate the correct treatment plan for the period of time before and after the procedure.

Endobiogenic clinical phytotherapy

Table 10. Plants effecting the corticotropic axis[25,27]

Plant	Form used	Action
Lavandula angustifolia	Essential oil, tincture, fluid extract, infusion	Central nervous system sedative, α-sympatholytic, β-sympatholytic, vagolytic, GABA-ergic, arterial dilatator
Melilotus officinalis	Tincture, fluid extract, Infusion	Central nervous system sedative and alphasympatholytic
Passiflora incarnate	Tincture, Fluid extract, infusion	Alphasympatholytic, sedative without causing somnolence, GABA-ergic, anxiolytic
Crataegus oxyacantha	Tincture, fluid extract, gemmo, infusion	Neurotropic, central nervous system sedative, strong a-sympatholytic

(Continued)

Table 10. (Continued)

Plant	Form used	Action
Ribes nigrum	Gemmo, fluid extract, tincture, infusion	Buds: betasympathomimetic, glucocorticoid stimulant. Leaves: glucocorticoid, anti-allergic, *betasympathomimetic*
Rosa canina	Gemmo, fluid extract	Adrenal cortex stimulant, *betasympathomimetic*
Satureja montana	Essential oil, fluid extract	Adrenal cortex stimulant (general), improves permissive cortisol
Sequoia gigantica	Gemmo	Dr Duraffourd mentions this plants ability as: 'adrenal cortex stimulant *favouring adrenal androgens and increasing DHEA*'; Reduces ACTH by classical inhibition
Thymus vulgaris	Essential oil, fluid extract, tincture, infusion	Adrenal cortex stimulant (essential oil form only)
Cinnamomum zeylanicum	Essential oil, fluid extract, tincture, decoction, infusion	Adrenal cortex stimulant, favouring glucocorticoids (Essential oil only)
Eleutherococcus senticosus	Decoction, fluid extract, tincture	Glucocorticoid stimulant
Glycyrrhiza glabra	Tincture, fluid extract, decoction	Potentiates effects of corticosteroids

Serotonin

Serotonin will be discussed in this section as it effects the HPA axis. It is believed that serotonin effects the HPA axis by 'regulating upstream corticotropin-releasing hormone (CRH) signalling systems in the paraventricular nucleus of the hypothalamus (PVH)'.[63] It is interesting to note that more than 90% of serotonin is made and stored in the intestines.[64]

In endobiogenic medicine, serotonin is seen as central para. As described by Dr's Lapraz and Hedayat:

> Acetylcholine also stimulates serotonin, which participates in the entrainment of neurotransmitters in the following fashion: Serotonin-dopamine-TRH-histamine-serotonin.[50]

Serotonin, centrally, initiates the process, which puts into place the metabolic activity that is responsible for learning, memory, planning etc. Serotonin can be described as the insulin of the brain, in so much as it facilitates the transfer of glucose across the blood-brain barrier.[50]

Serotonin also has clear peripheral activity linked to para. Peripherally, it is involved in the control of urination, as it regulates parasympathetic neural input to the bladder as well as somatic input to the external urinary sphincter. The effects of serotonin on the intestine are to control peristalsis, motility and intestinal secretions.[65] High peripheral serotonin increases the activity of the parasympathetic system and in so doing, increases congestion. This can diminish transport to the brain so central serotonin may decrease.[66]

A mechanism of low central serotonin

In stress states, the release of adrenalin and cortisol act to inhibit insulin. This is in order to spare the glucose generated for use by the vital organs, e.g. heart and brain. At this point, peripheral serotonin also plays a crucial role in this process. It too delays the activity of insulin. Central serotonin, however, acting as the insulin of the brain, facilitates the transfer of glucose into the brain. However, if the stress becomes chronic, central serotonin downregulates in order to prevent the brain from becoming overexposed to glucose which can be toxic.[50,66]

Endobiogenic clinical phytotherapy

Table 11. Plants effecting serotonin levels[25,67–69]

Plant	Form used	Action
Agrimonia eupeptoria	Tincture, fluid extract, Infusion	Serotonin regulator
Griffonia simplicifolia	Capsule	Contains 5-HTP (serotonin precursor), antidepressant, anti-anxiety, anti-panic, anti-insomnia
Rhodiola rosea	Tincture, fluid extract, decoction	Serotonergic, noradrenergic, dopaminergic, cholinergic, antidepressant, memory enhancement

CHAPTER NINE

Gonadotropic axis

T he gonadotropic axis is an anabolic axis, and it initiates metabolism. It also manages the genital hormones, which play a key role in the anabolism of proteins through their activity on the nuclei of the cells, thus contributing to cellular growth and the development of the muscles and bone.[50,72]

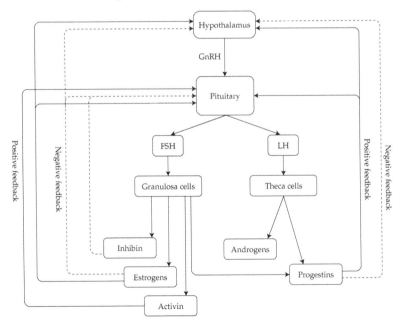

Figure 13. Hypothalamus–pituitary–gonadal axis in females.

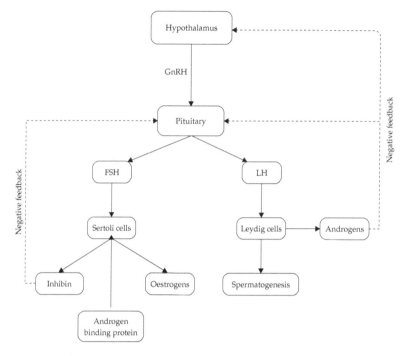

Figure 14. Hypothalamus–pituitary–gonadal axis in males.
- GnRH (gonadotropin-releasing hormone)
- FSH (follicle-stimulating hormone)
- LH (luteinising hormone)

FSH

FSH is secreted from the anterior pituitary gland and stimulates oestrogen production and secretion. It is necessary for fertility in both men and women.[70] FSH is equally important in men as well as women, not just for fertility but for the reasons that will be discussed now.

Cellular metabolism

As FSH is responsible for stimulating oestrogen production and secretion, it plays a vital role in initiating cellular metabolism at the level of transcription.[50]

Colon

There is a relatively greater number of FSH receptors in relation to LH receptors located on the right side of the body. In relation to the colon, there is a greater quantity of FSH receptors towards the right side of the transverse colon and in the ascending colon. See Figure 18, Chapter 12. The absorption of protein occurs at these locations under the influence of FSH.[71]

FSH makes oestrogen more active at a cellular level by upregulating oestrogen receptors. There are different scenarios for high FSH states. One example being a drop in peripheral oestrogen activity that can occur at specific times in a patient's life. This will result in an increase in FSH secretion and activity. In endobiogenic medicine, FSH is seen to be the structural initiator of autoimmune disease.[71]

High FSH activity can result in mucosal congestion of the colon, with the specific regions of the colon mentioned above being more vulnerable. When there is congestion, there is stagnation, and this affects the mucosa, thus participating in the development of Crohn's and colitis. As discussed in the section of drainage, the congestive phenomenon can ensue, as a result of an increased demand for nutrients by the organ in question. If this congestion is prolonged, it can become a factor in the disease process.[50]

LH

LH is secreted from the anterior pituitary and stimulates the synthesis and secretion of progesterone and testosterone.[73] In women LH stimulates androgen production in the thecal cells. In males, LH stimulates the Leydig cells of the testes to produce testosterone. Progesterone is also produced in the Leydig cells.[73]

Colon

There is a relatively greater number of LH receptors in relation to FSH receptors located on the left side of the body. In relation to the colon, there is a greater quantity of LH receptors towards the left side of the transverse colon and down the descending colon. See Figure 18, Chapter 12. The absorption of protein occurs at these locations under the influence of LH.[72]

Oestrogen

The feminising hormone. Oestrogen is an anabolic steroid hormone which plays an important role in fertility and gametogenesis in both men and women.[50] In females, oestrogens are produced in the granulosa cells of the ovaries. In men, oestrogens are produced in the Sertoli cells of the testicles.[74] In addition to gonadic production of oestrogen, there are also extra-gonadal sites of oestrogen production such as the adrenal glands and adipose tissue.[75,76] Of all sex steroids, oestrogen requires the greatest number of metabolic conversations, being derived from cholesterol as follows:

Cholesterol—progesterone—androgens—oestrogens

From an endobiogenic perspective, oestrogen plays a significant role in the initiation of protein metabolism for the construction of cells. However, it is androgens that complete the anabolic cycle of construction.[50]

The role of oestrogen and its various metabolites is a complex one, to say the least, and the measurement of serum levels of oestrogens do not yield adequate information of what is actually occurring at a cellular level. We discussed something similar earlier, when we spoke about the dysfunction that can occur in the HPA axis with regards to cortisol, and the same is true here. Serum levels of oestrogen may be elevated, but its activity on a cellular level may be low, or serum levels may be low, but for various reasons the little oestrogen there is, may be highly active at a cellular level. It is for these reasons that Drs Duraffourd and Lapraz developed the functional biology test used in endobiogenic medicine, where serum levels of these hormones are not evaluated, but rather the cellular and tissular activity is, as well as the relative activity between one and another.

Oestrogens effects on pathogens

Oestrogen exhibits profound effects on the intracellular environment of the organism by increasing the activity of viruses, bacteria and fungi. In the case of viruses, the increase of oestrogenic activity at a cellular level facilitates viral transcription by increasing intra-nuclear activity, such as the rate of DNA transcription. This is especially important to remember in hepatitis, as the development, intensity and duration of the virus is dependent on the level of oestrogen activity.[77]

Oestrogen and autoimmunity

Several studies have shown a connection between oestrogen and a variety of autoimmune diseases, including IBD. Oestrogens have both stimulatory and inhibitory effects on the immune system, as well as pro-inflammatory and anti-inflammatory effects.[78,79]

High levels of oestrogen have been shown to predispose patients to systemic lupus erythematosus (SLE) and to exacerbate active SLE. The mechanism is related to defective control of T-cell apoptosis induced by oestrogen, which is believed to allow for the persistence of autoreactive T-cells.[80] Furthermore, an abnormal oestrogen metabolism has been found to be present in both men and women with SLE, and there appears to be an imbalance in the ratio of oestrogen to testosterone with a bias towards oestrogen. It is believed that this imbalance places a crucial role in the immune dysfunction seen.[81]

The low androgen to estrogen ratio is significant in both sexes, and this is not specific to SLE. Indeed, low serum levels of both gonadal and adrenal androgens have been detected in both men and women with rheumatoid arthritis (RA). Androgens have been found to suppress autoimmunity by inhibiting peripheral blood mononuclear cell activity. In relation to RA, and again this is relevant in both sexes, the ratio of oestrogens to androgens in the Synovial Fluid is significantly elevated.[82]

With regards to the immune and inflammatory regulative effects of oestrogens; most of these effects are mediated by two oestrogen receptors (ERα and ERβ). These receptors can be found in a variety of cells, including immune cells, thus depending on which receptor is more active, will determine whether or not there will be an anti-inflammatory or pro-inflammatory outcome. With regards to IBD, reduced ERβ mRNA expression and increased gut permeability in animal studies was found to precede the onset of colitis.[83] In human studies, Looijer-van Langen et al. observed decreased ERβ mRNA levels in colonic biopsies of IBD patients.[84] Furthermore, a study involving 48 patients with IBD showed a significant increase of ERα and a decrease of ERβ activity in T lymphocytes.[83]

The role that oestrogen plays in autoimmunity is complex, and oestrogens have both stimulatory and inhibitory effects on the immune system.[78] This makes unravelling the mystery that oestrogen plays in the autoimmune process challenging. As discussed previously, in endobiogenic terms it is a question of relativity and the effect that these hormones have on a cellular level. For example, a drop in oestrogen can elicit a reactional increase in FSH, which augments the effects of oestrogen on a cellular level. This brings us back to the point that serum levels of hormones, in this example oestrogen, are not a good indicator of hormone activity and a low serum oestrogen level could actually mean a high cellular activity or a normal or high serum level of oestrogen could mean a low cellular activity. This, coupled with the modifications in other endocrine axes, could be enough to trigger autoimmunity.

In such a complex scenario, the evaluation of the functional biology indexes is crucial in assessing each autoimmune patient in order to determine which pathways are most effected within that specific patient.

Thyroid

Oestrogen increases the sensitivity of the anterior pituitary to TRH.[85] Oestrogen relaunches the thyroid as it is a growth hormone and needs metabolic activity to conduct growth.

Bone

The structure of the bones are directly related to oestrogens activity, and if there is a problem with the bones, there will be a problem along the gonadotropic axis that must be identified and treated.[72]

Oestrogens diminish extracellular calcium levels as they concentrate calcium within the bones; as a result, they favour spasmodic states. Androgens, having the opposite effect have an antispasmodic action.[50]

Androgens

The masculinising hormone. Androgens are anabolic steroid hormones produced by the testes in the Leydig cells and in the Theca cells of the ovaries. Androgens are also made in the adrenal glands.[86] Androgens have been found to suppress autoimmunity by inhibiting peripheral blood mononuclear cell activity.[82] Androgens play a significant role in metabolism. It is the androgens that complete the anabolic cycle.

This can be seen in a definitive way when a person stops growing in height. It is the androgens that close the epiphyseal plates and stop the growth. With regards to the reconstruction efforts of the organism, catabolic and anabolic activity is a day to day occurrence. If this process proceeds smoothly, then the organism will function well but, in many conditions, dysfunction can occur at this level. Crohn's disease is an example, and there can be a shift towards a net catabolic state. This is linked to a relatively low testosterone to oestrogen ratio, which can be seen in the biology of functions. Correcting this imbalance is crucial in the treatment of Crohn's disease.

Progesterone

Progesterone is a steroid hormone. In female's progesterone is made in the ovaries and in males in the testes. Progesterone is also synthesised in the adrenal glands.[87] In females, it plays a vital role in ovulation and pregnancy and in males it influences spermiogenesis.[88] Progesterone receptors are present in the gallbladder.[89] Progesterone's effect here is to inhibit contraction of the smooth muscle fibres of the gallbladder and acts to reduce gall bladder motricity.[31]

Progesterone has an important anti-autoimmune action by 'stimulating the Th2 responses and suppressing the differentiation of Th1 and Th17 cells'.[82] This is why many women can experience remission of their autoimmune condition while pregnant.

Endobiogenic clinical phytotherapy

Table 12. Plants effecting the gonadotropic axis[25,90]

Plant	Form used	Action
Lithspermum officinale	Mother tincture	Antigonadotropic: FSH and LH antagonist
Vitex agnus-castus	Tincture, fluid extract	Inhibits FSH, inhibits oestrogen uptake at peripheral receptors

(Continued)

Table 12. (Continued)

Plant	Form used	Action
Borago officinalis	Tincture, infusion	Antigonadotropic (inhibits FSH > LH)
Pygeum africanum	Mother tincture, microspheres, dried extract	Inhibits LH, prostate and pelvic decongestant
Mediacago sativa	Leaf	Oestrogenic, inhibits LH, anti-androgenic, contains provitamin K, uterine anti-haemorrhagic
Angelica archangelica	Essential oil, tincture, fluid extract, decoction	Oestrogenic, inhibits FSH
Avena sativa	Tincture, fluid extract, infusion of aerial parts, decoction of seeds	Oestrogenic
Foeniculum vulgare	Essential oil, decoction, fluid extract, tincture	Oestrogenic, emmenagogue
Menyanthes trifoliata	Tincture, fluid extract, infusion	Oestrogenic, anti-androgenic
Salvia officinalis	Essential oil, tincture, fluid extract, infusion	Oestrogenic
Eleuthrococcus senticosus	Tincture, fluid extract, decoction	Testicular androgen stimulant, oestrogenic
Panax quinquefolium	Tincture, fluid extract, decoction	Stimulates testicular androgen production, Oestrogenic
Zingiber officinale	Essential oil, decoction, tincture, fluid extract, dried extract	Stimulant of testicular androgens
Alchemilla vulgaris	Tincture, fluid extract, dried extract	Progesterone-like luteotropic activity with secondary inhibition of LH, pelvic decongestant
Achillea millefolium	Tincture, fluid extract, essential oil, infusion	Progesterone-like without inhibiting LH

CHAPTER TEN

Thyrotropic axis

The thyrotropic axis is a catabolic axis, and it mobilises energy reserves by increasing basic metabolism. As with all the vertical axis, there is interaxial communication, and the thyrotropic axis interacts with the somatotropic axis in order to co-ordinate reconstruction.

Catabolic function

The role of the thyroid is to support catabolism in order to provide all the material that the organism requires for anabolic reconstruction. At the level of the bones, the thyroid dismantles the structure of the bone in order to release calcium, which will then participate in the osteoblastic reconstruction.[91]

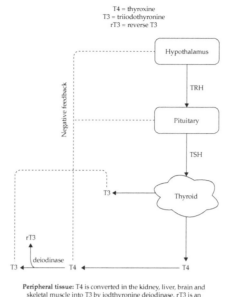

Figure 15. Hypothalamic–pituitary–thyroid axis.

TRH

- Secreted by the hypothalamus
- TRH is central beta
- TRH is stimulated by alphasympathetic activity

Actions of TRH

In endobiogenic medicine, TRH is seen as central beta. This is because TRH acts as a neuromodulator and increases the activity within the central nervous system.[50] Studies have shown that the actions of TRH are not restricted to its vertical axis, as seen in its role in the thyrotropic axis; that it exhibits extra thyrotropic axial activity.[92] TRH has also been found to be present in the gastrointestinal tract, pancreatic β cells and reproductive tracts.[93]

   TRH is implicated in psychiatric disorders. A consistent blunted response to TRH stimulation has been found in depressive patients. Within the field of biological psychiatry, a diminished TSH response to TRH administration has been established as one of the most reproducible findings.[94] Abnormal TRH levels have also been observed in Schizophrenic patients.[95] This abnormal TRH activity is recognised in endobiogenic medicine, as in schizophrenia, it is not a simple question of a solely abnormal dopamine activity. An increase in TRH activity is linked to ruminations, obsessive-compulsive disorder, anxiety and panic attack, as it increases the activity of the mind. TRH can also disrupt the normal rhythm of sleep and can stimulate the mind resulting in colourful and vivid dreams and nightmares.[50]

TRH plays a role in glucoregulation. It has the ability to stimulate the endocrine pancreas to secrete insulin and glucagon.[96,97]

Changes with the season

TRH rises in the autumn time, as the thyroid has to increase its activity to deal with the greater metabolic demands of winter.

TSH

TSH is produced and secreted by the thyrotrophs in the anterior pituitary gland. T3, T4, somatostatin, dopamine and glucocorticoids all inhibit TSH.[93] TSH also exhibits extra thyroid activity, and TSH receptors have been found in various other tissues in the body.[98]

Actions of TSH

TSH is involved in the regulation of bone density, and TSH receptors are found in osteoblasts and osteoclasts.[99] In endobiogenic medicine, the thyroid is seen to play a role in all types of autoimmune disease and not just autoimmune disease of the thyroid. It is also implicated in inflammation.[91] An increase in circulating thyroid hormone (TH) has been linked to an increase in the pro-inflammatory activity of specific immune cells. Namely, neutrophil, macrophage and dendritic cells. It is believed that the pro-inflammatory mechanism of TH is linked to its functional intracellular metabolism. Oxidative stress is another mechanism by which thyroid hormones are implicated in inflammation. Both hyperthyroidism and hypothyroidism are linked to an increase in oxidative stress, but for different reasons. In hyperthyroidism there is an increase in reactive oxygen species and in hypothyroidism there is a decrease in antioxidant status.[100]

As well as its role in inflammation, TH also plays an important role in the defence of the organism by assisting in the modulation of the innate immune system.[101] In fact, a higher level of T3 and T4, but within normal physiological levels has been shown to enhance both innate and adaptive immunity by effecting the activity of a variety of immune cells, which include, natural killer cells, lymphocytes, monocytes and macrophages.[102,103] Dysfunctions in these pathways are linked to a variety of conditions including autoimmune disease, inflammation and viral infections.[103]

Endobiogenic clinical phytotherapy

Table 13. Plants effecting the thyrotropic axis[25,104,105,106]

Plant	Form used	Action
Avena sativa	Tincture, fluid extract, decoction of seed, infusion of aerial parts	Thyroid stimulant (T4, T3), reduces TSH by feedback regulation
Brassica napus	Mother tincture	Thyroid antagonist
Fabiana imbricata	Mother tincture	TRH antagonist
Leonurus cardiaca	Tincture, fluid extract, infusion	TRH antagonist, TSH antagonist
Lycopus europaeus	Tincture	Antigonadotropic, central thyroid antagonist (TSH>TRH), inhibits the transformation of T4 to T3, diminishes the peripheral effects of thyroid hormones
Melissa officinalis	Essential oil, tincture, fluid extract, infusion	Inhibits TSH

CHAPTER ELEVEN

Somatotropic axis

The somatotropic axis is an anabolic axis and manages the cellular development of the organism through the activity of growth hormone, which increases the speed of synthesis of proteins and other cell elements.

The somatotropic axis plays an important role in the general adaptation syndrome. Its role here is to facilitate the reconstruction of the organism in order to maintain the initial state of functioning. The thyrotropic and gonadotropic axes are also involved in this activity, as the gonadotropic axis will provide the raw material needed for reconstruction and the thyrotropic axis, the fuel for this construction.

The role of the pancreas here, is essential in supporting cellular growth and development through the actions of insulin, which reduces blood glucose levels and facilitates the transfer of glucose into the cells and the release of glucagon which ultimately acts to raise blood glucose levels.[107]

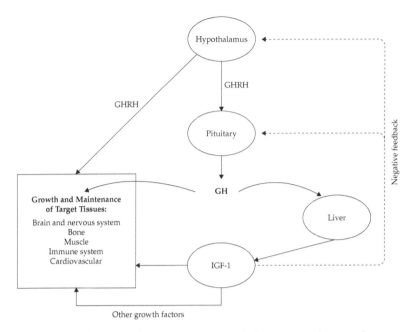

Figure 16. The anabolic cascade. GHRH = Growth hormone-releasing hormone; GH = Growth hormone.

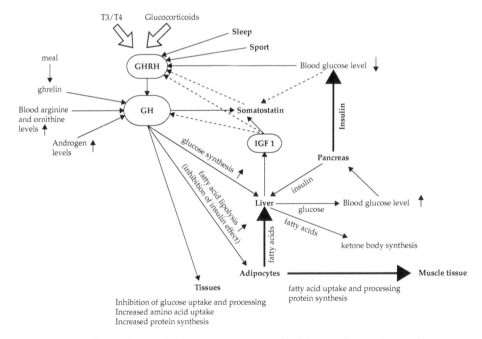

Figure 17. The effect of growth hormone (GH) on the blood glucose level. (T_3 = triiodo-thyronine, T_4 = thyroxine, GH = growth hormone, IGF-1 = insulin-like growth factor 1, GHRH = Growth hormone-releasing hormone. Broken arrow = inhibition; thin solid arrow = stimulation, large white arrow = permissive role).

Growth hormone

Growth hormone (GH) is synthesised in the pituitary gland by the somatotropic cells. Growth hormone-releasing hormone (GHRH) stimulates the synthesis and release of GH and somatostatin inhibits it. There are many other factors that govern the stimulation and inhibition of GH. Oestrogen, ghrelin, dopamine, TSH, hypoglycaemia and alphasympathetic activity, all stimulate GH. Insulin-like growth factor (IGF-1), insulin and cortisol inhibit GH. However, GHRH and somatostatin have the most pronounced effect on GH.[93, 108]

Functions of GH

GH stimulates the production of IGF-1 in the liver and these two growth factors both effect the growth of the muscles, bone and cartilage.[108] GH stimulates gluconeogenesis and glycogenolysis from the liver and kidney and in so doing raises blood glucose levels in order to provide energy. GH also has the effect of inducing insulin resistance.[109]

GH stimulates lipolysis, which results in an increase in the circulation of free fatty acids. These free fatty acids provide a valuable source of energy which is needed for the construction of the cells and tissues of the organism. The increase in circulating free fatty acids also contributes to insulin resistance.[109] GH also, increases the absorption of amino acids from the intestinal lumen, which as well as providing a source of energetic substrate provides material for the use of construction of the gut mucosa, as well as the other tissues in the body, especially the muscles.[110]

Prolactin

Most people, when thinking of prolactin, think about its role in lactation and breast tissue development. Prolactin's role in the organism, however, is much more diverse and effects metabolism as well as immunity. Dopamine, somatostatin and progesterone all inhibit prolactin and TRH, oestrogen, alphasympathetic activity and suckling stimulate prolactin.[111–113] Here, we can see another example of how the different hormonal axis cross communicates with each other, working as a whole in the management of the organism.

Prolactin is produced in the anterior part of the pituitary gland. However, prolactin can also be synthesised in various other regions of the body outside of the pituitary gland. These regions include the brain, ovaries, decidua, mammary glands, prostate, adipose tissue as well as lymphocytes.[114]

Prolactin acts as a hormone and also as a cytokine.[114] Prolactin regulates the immune system and modulates the function of both T- and B-cells.[115] Research has demonstrated that oestrogens stimulatory effect on autoreactive B-cells is dependent on prolactin. As mentioned, lymphocytes are also capable of producing prolactin, and its function here is to act as an autocrine or paracrine mediator.[116]

Animal studies have found that stress-induced prolactin release is a factor that is linked to intestinal inflammation. This occurs, as prolactin causes a dysfunction in

T-cell activity and an alteration in dendritic cells (DC) triggering them to produce the inflammatory mediators IL-6 and IL-23.[117]

Insulin

Insulin is produced in the endocrine pancreas by the beta cells in the islets of Langerhans. Insulin has an effect on all the tissues in the organism either directly or indirectly.[93] It is the hypoglycaemiant hormone and as such regulates the glucose entry into the cells which is generated by gluconeogenesis and glycogenolysis or obtained from dietary origin.

The level of circulating glucose is only one of the factors that trigger the release of insulin. TRH, prolactin, glucagon and vagal stimulation will also increase insulin secretion, and somatostatin inhibits its secretion.[93,96,97,118,119]

As we discussed earlier in the book, centrally it is not insulin but serotonin that facilitates the transfer of glucose into the cells. Centrally insulin has a different effect. It functions as a neuromodulator and plays a role in memory and learning.[120]

From an endobiogenic perspective, the endocrinometabolic effects of insulin are crucial in understanding its role in disease, and insulin does more than reduce blood glucose.

Insulin is involved in the energy supply and maintenance of the somatotropic axis. Insulin is involved, at every level and every stage, in the construction of the organism and its maintenance, hence it can be seen as the functional architect. It is a major cause of tissular inflammation, contributing to all types of inflammatory diseases. Furthermore, insulin has been found to significantly increase free radical production.[107,121–124]

Endobiogenic clinical phytotherapy

Table 14. Plants effecting the somatotropic axis[25]

Plant	Form used	Action
Fragaria vesca	Mother tincture	Reduces growth hormone and prolactin
Poterium sanguisorba	Mother tincture	Inhibits growth hormone and prolactin
Juglans regia	Mother tincture	Hypoglycemiant; reduces insulin resistance
Agrimonia eupeptoria	Tincture, fluid extract, infusion	Hypoglycemiant; reduces insulin resistance
Malva sylvestris	Mother tincture, tincture, infusion	Hyperglycemiant; reduces the effects of insulin on the cells. *Malva sylvestris* increases insulin resistance

Now that we have examined all four endocrine axes, it is possible to see how in a clinical setting, one cannot purely treat one axis or address a single hormone imbalance without understanding the role of the other axes in the disturbance.

For example, in the case of hypothyroidism, it is not advisable to simply push the function of the thyroid gland without understanding the true aetiology of the condition and thus the involvement of the other axes. To do so can be detrimental to the organism.

As well as vertical axes, there also exist horizontal axes which interconnect the four vertical axes. Figure 18 gives a simple illustration of this. In-depth evaluation of the horizontal axes will be reserved for other endobiogenic material as it is beyond the scope of this book.

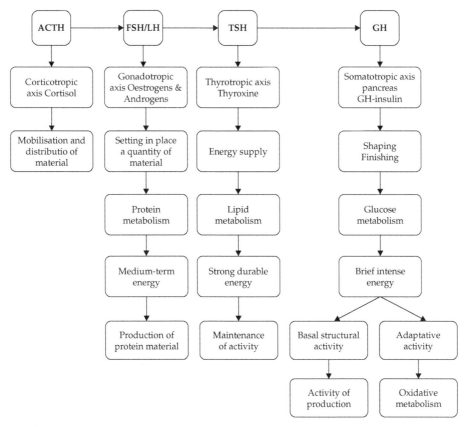

Figure 18. Endocrine system as 'the manager'.

CHAPTER TWELVE

The microbiome of the gut

The microbiome of the digestive system can be defined as the sum total of the different bacterial populations inhabiting the length of the digestive tract.

The bacterial species of the gut can be divided into the following categories:

- Beneficial flora
- Pathogenic flora
- Transient flora

The microbiome of the gut is a true intestinal ecosystem. The sheer diversity of bacterial species inhabiting the human gut is remarkable, with approximately 150–200 common species and about 1000 less common species.[125] While the microbiota consists largely of bacteria, there are also viruses, protozoa, archaea and fungi present, which are part of the intestinal ecosystem, having co-evolved with human beings.[125]

The microbiota is of vital importance and essential for not only the health of the digestive system but also the health of the entire organism. These microbes are involved in the digestion of complex indigestible polysaccharides and the synthesis of vitamins—all hydrosoluble vitamins (B1, B2, B6, PP (nicotinic acid), B5, H (biotin), folic acid and B12), except vitamin C, liposoluble vitamins (K)—and assist in the inhibition of pathogens.[127] In addition to this, the gut microbiota contributes to the production of bile acids, choline and short-chain fatty acids (SCFA).[125] SCFA are produced in the gut by the fermentation of carbohydrates and proteins and provide a valuable source of energy to the organism as well as supporting the growth of beneficial gut flora.

Efficient synthesis of SCFA production has been linked to a reduced risk of developing several chronic illnesses.[135]

Disturbances in a healthy microbiome of the gastrointestinal system have been linked to disease in all ages.[134] As we will see, this includes Irritable bowel syndrome (IBS) and IBD.

The gut–brain connection

It is interesting that the microbes in the gut are approximately the same weight as the human brain, weighing in at 1 kg. It is believed that these microbes have played an important role in the development of the brain, affecting behaviour and cognitive function. In fact, there has been much research in recent years focusing on the connection between the gut and the brain, which is called the brain–gut-microbiota axis. This is a bi-directional axis. Involved in this axis are the neuroendocrine and neuro-immune systems, the central nervous system, the entire autonomic nervous system (para, alpha and beta), the enteric nervous system and the intestinal microbiota.[125]

The microbes of the gastrointestinal system are capable of producing several neurotransmitters and neuromodulators. Certain Lactobacillus and Bifidobacterium species produce GABA. *Escherichia*, *Bacillus* and *Saccharomyces* spp. produce noradrenaline, with *Bacillus* also producing dopamine. Lactobacilli produce acetylcholine. *Candida*, *Streptococcus*, *Escherichia* and *Enterococcus* spp. produce 5-HTP.[125] Approximately 95% of the serotonin in the body is produced in the gut, largely by the enterochromaffin cells of the mucosa.[129]

Dysbiosis of the gut has been linked to a variety of mental health problems and a recent clinical study involving the administration of two types of probiotics (*Lactobacillus helveticus* R0052 and *Bifidobacterium longum* R0175) given simultaneously for 30 days showed a significant improvement compared to controls in the Hospital Anxiety and Depression Scale and in the Hopkins Symptoms Checklist.[126] Furthermore, in the same study, the probiotic combination was prescribed to a group of patients with the lowest urinary free cortisol, of which levels were less than 50 ng/ml at baseline. Improvements in anxiety levels, obsessive-compulsive behaviour and paranoid ideations were seen.[126]

The microbiota and the HPA axis

It has become evident that the microbiota of the gastrointestinal system can affect the activity of the HPA axis as well as the immune response. The question is, how is the microbiota affecting the central activity of the organism?[129]

There seems to be a complex bi-directional communication system along the brain–gut-microbiota axis. The microbiota can cause changes peripherally and along the CNS by stimulating cytokine production, neuropeptide and neurotransmitter release and by affecting the vagus nerve. The signals generated are capable of crossing the blood-brain barrier where they influence the activity of the microglia. The microglia play an important role in immune surveillance, synaptic pruning and clearance of debris as well as affecting the HPA axis regulation state. Due to the effect on the HPA axis, glucocorticoids are secreted, which in turn help regulate microglial function.[129,139] These glucocorticoids also influence cytokine release, as well as the trafficking of monocytes from the spleen to the brain.[129,140]

Owing to the complex effects produced by the microbiota, it is now seen to play a major role in the phenomenon of stress adaptation. It is believed that dysbiosis of the gut can affect the organism's ability to adapt appropriately to stress and to regulate the immune system correctly. What is also important here is the actual diversity of the micro-organisms present within the gut.[129]

The mechanism of how stress negatively affects the gut is related to the HPA axis. As we know, CRH secretion induced by a stressor triggers the release of ACTH and ACTH triggers the release of cortisol from the adrenal cortex. What is relevant here, on a gastrointestinal level, is that animal studies have shown that CRH stimulates the release of pro-inflammatory cytokines TNFa, IL1b and IL6, which affect the bowels.[133] In human studies, research shows that TNFa, in particular, affects the epithelial lining of the bowel by altering the structure and function of the tight junction.[136] This is commonly seen in Crohn's disease. From a treatment perspective, the probiotic *Lactobacillus farciminis*, when fed to mice, reduced the intestinal permeability of the bowel. The publication quotes; *'This highlights the two-way nature of the HPA axis and our resident gut microbiota'*.[133]

IBS and the microbiota

IBS can severely affect quality of life with symptoms including abdominal pain, bloating, constipation and diarrhoea.[137] Even though the aetiology and presentation of IBS is very different to that of IBD, inflammation is still present.

A study involving 151 subjects 76 patients and 75 controls showed that the levels of cortisol and the pro-inflammatory cytokines IL6 and IL8 were elevated in the IBS patients. A positive correlation between a rise in ACTH and IL6 was observed.[133] Several types of Lactobacilli and Bifidobacterium probiotics have been found to normalise corticosterone and ACTH plasma levels. These same probiotics also act to reduce CRH, IL6 and TNFa.[138] Once again, we can see that there is bi-directional communication at play. The gut microbiota is capable of inducing hormonal changes which can result in inflammation, and hormones themselves can affect the gut, affecting the composition of the microbiota.[134]

Dysbiosis and IBD

Specific strains of micro-organisms, including Escherichia and Fusobacterium, have been found to reside in the gut of IBD sufferers, with the potential to exacerbate inflammation and/or invade intestinal epithelial cells.[130] *Rothia mucilaginosa* was also found to be present at increased levels in patients with intestinal ulcer formation.

Rothia mucilaginosa is an opportunistic pathogen present in immunocompromised patients.[141] Most of these organisms are generally present in the oral and upper respiratory tract where they comprise part of the normal microbiota. They are, however, relatively rare in the colon and when present signify dysbiosis. These micro-organisms can begin to colonise the colon in states of disturbed mucosal barrier function.[130] With regards to oral dysbiosis present in Crohn's disease, the micro-organisms Haemophilus and Veillonella have been found to be present in the oral cavity of these patients.[130]

A terrain within the gastrointestinal system which favours a less diverse microbiome has been consistently linked to the development of IBD.[142–145] The largest single cohort microbiome study, involving newly diagnosed paediatric patients, identified significant mucosal dysbiosis at early disease stage. These patients had not yet undergone any treatment. Patients with a variety of disease phenotypes with respect to location, severity, and behaviour were included. Furthermore, the study combined two additional cohorts with the risk cohort, resulting in a total of 1742 samples from paediatric or adult patients with either new-onset or established disease.[132]

Evaluation of the microbiome samples revealed that the inflammation present in Crohn's disease was found to be linked to a reduction in the overall number of different species of microbes. '*Disease status correlated strongly with an increased abundance of Enterobacteriaceae, Pasteurellacaea, Veillonellaceae, and Fusobacteriaceae and decreased abundance of Erysipelotrichales, Bacteroidales, and Clostridiales*'.[132]

Genetic studies propose that Crohn's patients do not have the ability to correctly manage the environment of their intestines. Patients are unable to either cultivate beneficial flora or correctly manage the pathogenic or dysbiotic species.[147] In addition to this, medication such as antibiotics, which profoundly modify the environment of the gut, reducing the diversity of the micro-organisms, increase the risk of developing IBD.[132] What actually benefits the gut is an abundance of butyrate-producing bacteria, such as *Faecalibacterium prausnitzii* (clostridial cluster IV) and *Anaerostipes*, *Eubacterium* and *Roseburia* species (clostridial cluster XIVa), adequate branch chain amino acid biosynthesis and good antioxidant states. These factors have been found to be essential for the resolution of intestinal inflammation.[131,146]

Birth: a crucial time for the microbiome

The birthing process is a crucial time for the development of the microbiota, as infants are first exposed to microbes from the mother, and the mode of delivery plays a major part (vaginally born vs C-section). Vaginally delivered infants will benefit vastly by obtaining the micro-organisms from the birthing canal. This is when the very first seeding of the gastrointestinal system takes place.[148,149]

It is now believed that the microbes that populate our gut in early life influence our neural development via microglia activation. As such, disruptions (such as stress or antibiotic treatment) to our microbiota at this critical period of dynamic microbiota–host interactions have the potential to profoundly alter gut–brain signalling, affect health throughout life and increase the risk of neurodevelopmental disorders.[129]

The microbiota of infants is unstable and there is a low diversity of microbes at least for the first 2.5 years of life. At that point, the composition of the microbiota resembles that of an adult.[125] A good foundation in relation to the microbiome is essential for good health, both at the start of life and in later life as well. It is essential that the infant is given the best chance of developing a healthy gut flora. Studies show that full-term, breastfed, vaginally delivered and non-antibiotic treated infants have the best chances of developing a healthy gut flora.[128]

The microbiome and Immunity

In the gut, there is a symbiotic relationship between the microbiota and the mucosa of the bowel, which is essential for gut homeostasis. The gut is actually considered to be the largest immunological organ in the body and as such is able to regulate innate and adaptive immune responses.[178]

The gut mucosal immune system, which is dependent on a healthy microbiome, forms a protective barrier for the intestines. It consists of lymph nodes, lamina propria and epithelial cells.[179] Research has shown that when dysbiosis occurs, intestinal disease develops due to immune dysfunction.[179,181] Intestinal dysbioses has been shown to cause an abnormal adaptive immune response resulting in an increase in IBD inflammatory activity and damage to the gastrointestinal tract.[182] Indeed, loss of intestinal barrier function is necessary for autoimmunity to develop.[184]

Epithelial cells are reinforced by tight junctions, and it is these tight junctions that act as the main mechanical barrier of the intestinal mucosal surface, preventing microbial contamination of the interstitial tissues. A loss of integrity of the tight junction structure can be a result of a dysfunction in the regulatory signals or a result of specific protein mutations. When this occurs, there is a breakdown in the homeostasis of the gut.[180]

It is interesting that evidence now shows that intestinal dysbiosis, loss of intestinal barrier function and environmental factors play a significant role in the development of IBD. Genetic susceptibility is not sufficient enough on its own to trigger IBD.[179,183]

Dysbiosis and its different forms

Definition: Dysbiosis is an imbalance in the growth and distribution of the different bacterial species within the gastrointestinal tract. Dysbiosis can be acute, chronic or latent.

Acute intestinal dysbiosis results in acute enterocolitis. This occurs due to overwhelming aggression by a pathogen against an organism that is in balance, but whose defence capabilities are temporarily overwhelmed. It can also be a result of a less intense aggression, against a marginally imbalanced organism, resulting in its acute decompensation.[178]

Chronic intestinal dysbiosis

Classically speaking, chronic dysbiosis is related to a number of gastrointestinal disorders where stasis is present. These conditions include: stenoses (as seen in Crohn's disease), intestinal diverticula, blind loops, surgical procedures (anastomoses) or suppression of the ileocecal valve, as well as illnesses causing loss of intestinal peristalsis, e.g. gastroparesis or scleroderma.

From an *endobiogenic perspective*: chronic dysbiosis is linked to upstream blockages in organic and neuroendocrine relationships. We have already discussed how dysfunctions in the HPA axis can affect the microbiome. We will look at this further in the next couple of chapters.[178]

Latent intestinal dysbiosis

Occurs due to periodic alterations in the microbiome. With

- An incipient dysbiosis that has not fully expressed itself and is limited to a particular part of the bowel.
- The possibility of decompensation if there is an aggression (external or internal). This may involve:
  - Chronic low-grade inflammation which results in leaky gut and as a result there is decreased nutrient absorption
  - Impaired host immunity against pathogenic organisms[178]

Variations in intestinal flora

From an endobiogenic perspective, the organism alters the flora of the intestines according to its metabolic needs. Because of this, bacteria-host and bacteria-bacteria interactions are dependent on

1. The age of the individual, which is related to their level of endobiogenic equilibrium.
2. Metabolic needs are secondary to the mechanisms of adaptation and adaptability, unique to each individual.
3. The immune mechanisms of adaptation that begin in the gut.[178]

This explains the considerable variation between one individual and another.

Upstream effects on intestinal mucosa

The mucosa of the gut is affected by upstream neuroendocrine changes, in an attempt to carefully select and absorb specific nutrients that are necessary for a particular metabolic need. This can be termed 'adaptive solicitation of the mucosa'. Hence, there is an increase in congestion of particular sections of the intestine, an increase in the nutrition of certain flora and a modification of the pH. These changes alter the mucosa of the intestines.

This causes changes in

a. the volume of various compartments of the gut
b. the structure of the gut wall
c. the absorbent surface of the mucosa

There is a global action favouring the growth of the intestinal mucosa.[178]

Autonomic nervous system factors

The autonomic nervous system and each of its subdivisions have specific effects on the digestive tract, as listed below. They alter the microbiome in various ways by affecting the function of the intestines and sphincters. When peristalsis is reduced, there is an increase in the contact time between the contents of the gut and the gut wall. When peristalsis is increased, there is less contact time between the contents of the gut and the gut wall. This will affect the microbiome in its own right.

Parasympathetic system

- stimulates bile secretion
- stimulates parotid and exocrine pancreatic secretions
- increases peristalsis

Alphasympathetic system

- increases congestion
- slows peristalsis
- closes sphincters, e.g. sphincter of Oddi

Betasympathetic system

- increases bile flow
- opens the sphincters[178]

Endocrine factors

From an endobiogenic perspective, the microbiome of the gut is regulated by the endocrine system. It has the ability to alter the microbiome, selecting specific flora that answer its particular metabolic needs.

It is able to achieve this by:

a) simply modifying the proportion of each of the microbial strains present.
b) affecting the distribution of the microbial strains along the gut.

A situation may be present, where there is a particular endocrine appeal that favours the selection of local saprophytic flora, which answer to the required metabolic activity. This may lead the organism to create an 'autoimmune' activity in order to neutralise certain microbes.

There are various receptors in specific locations of the large intestine. As seen in Figure 19, the receptors present are: ACTH, FSH, TRH, TSH, LH, PRL and GH. These receptors play a fundamental role in the phenomena of adaptation, both structural and adaptive. They play a compensatory role if the colon is solicited by adaptative phenomena—a situation that may lead to disease (e.g. Crohn's disease).[17]

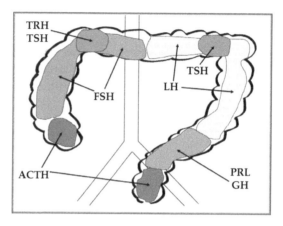

Figure 19. Receptor location in the colon (metabolic sequence).[70]

CHAPTER THIRTEEN

Treatment aimed at correcting the microbiome

R emember the four levels of treatment discussed earlier

1. symptomatic
2. drainage
3. treating at the level of the ANS
4. treating at the level of the endocrine system

Symptomatic level of treatment

First, it is important to correctly identify and treat any external aggravating factors, such as microbes in foods, dietary irritants (either specific to the patient or general to most patients) and remove foods that promote the growth of pathogenic gut flora and contribute to inflammation. This will be discussed in detail in the section on diet. Environmental toxins and medications can also participate in the modification of the microbiome, as discussed earlier.

Second, address internal factors such as distal sources of infection, e.g. ENT and dental infections that can be transported into the gut or place a burden on the organism.

At a symptomatic level, treatment should comprise of:

1. Antiseptic agents capable of killing the pathogenic gut flora.
2. Removal of the external agents responsible for causing the imbalance such as stress, lifestyle, diet and medication, such as, NSAIDs, hormonal therapies, antibiotics, PPI medications, etc.
3. Addressing the distal infection or infections if present. This may involve the treatment of or removal of an infected tooth, etc.

In cases of acute dysbiosis, it is common that the disorder becomes chronic.

With regards to drainage

It is important to assure good functioning of the emunctories. This can be achieved by draining the specific organs involved in the dysbiosis with chosen medicinal plants.

At the level of the autonomic nervous system

Treating at the level of the autonomic nervous system is essential in order to ensure good functioning of bile flow (bile ducts, gall bladder), pancreatic secretions and intestinal peristalsis. Make sure to treat any imbalances of the ANS, as discussed in previous chapters. Imbalances involving dysfunctions of alpha, para and beta.

At the level of the endocrine system

It is necessary to treat imbalances of the endocrine system that have been put in place by the organism for various reasons which will become apparent from the case history. These imbalances result in a programmed and repetitive endocrine appeal that causes a disruption of the microbiome through a selection of a particular flora.

Materia medica

Table 15. Bactericidal plants[25,150–159]

Plant	Form used	Part used
Vaccinium myrtillus	Decoction, infusion, gemmo, fluid extract, tincture, capsule	Berry, leaf
Rubus fruticosus	Gemmo, mother tincture, tincture, decoction, infusion	Shoots, leaf, fruit
Juglans regia	Mother tincture, tincture, decoction	Bark, hull, leaf
Origanum vulgare	Essential oil, capsule	Aerial parts
Allium sativum	Fluid extract, tincture, capsule, essential oil	Bulb
Cinnamomum zeylanicum	Essential oil, tincture, capsule	Leaf and bark

Table 16. Antispasmodic plants[25,160–166]

Plant	Form used	Part used
Viburnum opulus	Fluid extract, tincture, decoction, capsule	Root
Angelica archangelica	Fluid extract, tincture, decoction, capsule, essential oil	Root
Foeniculum vulgare	Fluid extract, tincture, decoction, capsule, essential oil	Seed
Glycyrrhiza glabra	Fluid extract, tincture, decoction, capsule	Root
Melissa officinalis	Fluid extract, tincture, essential oil, infusion, capsule	Leaf and stem
Matricaria chamomilla	Fluid extract, tincture, essential oil, infusion, capsule	Flower
Carum carvi	Fluid extract, tincture, decoction, essential oil, capsule	Seed

Plants acting on the autonomic nervous system

Table 17. Sympatholytic and parasympatholytic[25,27,167]

Plant	Form used	Part used
Angelica archangelica	Fluid extract, tincture, decoction, capsule, essential oil	Root
Levisticum officinale	Fluid extract, tincture, decoction, capsule, essential oil	Root, seed and leaf
Lavandula officinalis	Fluid extract, tincture, infusion, capsule, essential oil	Flower

Table 18. Parasympatholytic[25]

Plant	Form used	Part used
Thymus vulgaris: neurotropic antispasmodic	Essential oil, fluid extract, tincture, infusion, capsule	Aerial parts
Matricaria chamomilla: musculotropic and neurotropic antispasmodic	Fluid extract, tincture, essential oil, infusion, capsule	Flower
Artemisia dracunculus	Essential oil	Leaf

Table 19. Betasympathomimetic EO form only[25]

Plant	Form used	Part used
Cinnamomum zeylanicum	Essential oil	Leaf and bark
Satureja montana	Essential oil	Leaf and flower

Table 20. Laxative plants[25,27,168]

Plant	Form used	Part used
Althaea officinalis root	Decoction, infusion, tincture	Root, leaf, flower
Malva Sylvestris	Infusion, mother tincture	Flower
Plantago psyllium	Powder	Seed and husk
Rumex crispus	Decoction, tincture	Root

Table 21. Tannin-containing plants[25,27,168]

Plant	Form used	Part used
Agrimonia eupatoria	Infusion, tincture	Leaf, flower
Fragaria vesca	Infusion, mother tincture	Leaf, root
Juglans regia	Mother tincture	Leaf
Rubus fructicosus	Infusion, tincture	Leaf

Table 22. Anti-fungal and anti-parasitic plants[25,169-177]

Plant	Form used	Part used
Salvia officinalis	Essential oil, tincture, fluid extract, infusion, capsule	Leaf
Eugenia cariophyllata	Essential oil, fluid extract, tincture, capsule, decoction	Floral button and stems
Juglans regia	Mother tincture, tincture, decoction	Bark, Hull, Leaf
Cinnamomum zeylanicum	Essential oil, tincture, capsule	Leaf and bark
Thymus vulgaris	Essential oil, fluid extract, tincture, infusion, capsule	Aerial parts
Satureja montana	Essential oil	Leaf and flower

Green clay

This is a truly outstanding therapeutic agent. It has anti-infectious, anti-fungal, anti-inflammatory and detoxifying actions. Green clay will be discussed in detail later on in the book.

Probiotics to rebalance the intestinal flora

Probiotics should be taken as far away as possible from aromatic preparations as they will be damaged by them. In acute cases of dysbiosis, probiotic treatment should be continued for several days after the disappearance of symptoms.

Enzyme therapy

If there are signs of exocrine pancreatic insufficiency, it is necessary to support pancreatic activity. This can be done with the use of either systemic enzymes or digestive enzymes, depending on the case.

CHAPTER FOURTEEN

IBS, IBD and inflammation

N ow that you have a good understanding of the basic factors that govern the terrain, we can look at specific diseases and the mechanisms behind them. We need to understand in detail the mechanisms in order to treat our patients correctly.

When we talk about autoimmune activity, we are fundamentally talking about a chronic inflammatory state that is present in the organism and which is targeting a specific organ, group of organs or specific tissues. The inflammatory state is what causes the awful symptoms seen in these chronic conditions, especially in the case of IBD. We must evaluate and understand the cause of the inflammation present in order to treat the mechanism and not just the symptoms.

For the purposes of this book, we will be discussing the conditions know as IBS and IBD (Crohn's disease and ulcerative colitis).

Irritable bowel syndrome (IBS)

IBS is a chronic functional gastrointestinal disorder. Symptoms consist of abdominal pain or discomfort, bloating, diarrhoea and constipation. Fatigue is also a common symptom. IBS is not officially classified as a pathology, as there are no detectable structural and biochemical abnormalities present.[187,188]

There are many factors that have been implicated in the pathogenesis of IBS, amongst them are

- altered gastrointestinal motility
- visceral hypersensitivity

- intestinal inflammation
- post-infectious reactivity
- food sensitivity
- carbohydrate malabsorption
- brain-gut-microbiota interactions
- gastrointestinal dysbiosis[189]

Some physicians have suggested that IBS symptomatology is secondary to psychological disturbances and not of primary relevance.[187] Often, IBS patients can be regarded as neurotic and referred to as psychiatric cases. However, if we view IBS in this way, we would be ignoring the link between digestively active peptides and the endogenous peptides in the CNS which are responsible for the motor and secretory effects of the digestive tract. Furthermore, we would be disregarding the correct physiological function of the colon, which plays a major role in the adaptative capacities of the organism. The symptoms that manifest in the colon are a reflection of the imbalances of the organism as a whole.

Patients with IBS are highly susceptible and reactive to stressors, both psychological (in relation to the mobilisation of the general adaptation syndrome) and on an alimentary level (in relation to food substances). All of this demonstrates the importance of the digestive function in the adaptative compensation of the organism.[186]

Inflammatory bowel disease (IBD)

Crohn's disease (CD) and ulcerative colitis (UC)

Inflammatory bowel disease is now a global disease which is becoming increasingly more prevalent in newly industrialised countries that have become more Westernised. Incidence in Western countries seems to have stabilised, but the health care burden remains high.[190]

Crohn's disease: pathology

Crohn's disease is classified as a chronic inflammatory bowel disease characterised by mucosal ulceration and inflammation. The ulceration seen in CD may occur anywhere along the gastrointestinal tract but most commonly affects the distal small intestine. Chronic diarrhoea, pain in the right iliac fossa and wasting are common symptoms of CD.[191]

Distinguishing features include:

- Transmural inflammation involving the whole thickness of the bowel wall.
- Lesions are segmented. There are healthy areas of mucosa set between ulcerated regions.

- Inflammatory response associated with lymphoid aggregates and granulomas (in 50–60% of patients).
- The small bowel can become thickened and narrowed.
- Ulcers/fissures in the mucosa.
- Possibly fistulae/abscesses in the colon.[191,192]

Ulcerative colitis: pathology

Ulcerative colitis is a chronic inflammatory disease involving ulceration of the colonic mucosa. UC affects the most distal part of the intestine, starting from the rectum and covering a greater or lesser portion of the distal descending colon. It is most often characterised by bloody diarrhoea.

Distinguishing features include:

- Inflamed mucosa which bleeds easily.
- Inflammation is superficial unlike Crohn's disease.
- Chronic inflammatory cells infiltrate the lamina propria.
- Extensive ulceration affecting the mucosa and submucosa. The muscularis is only affected in severe disease.
- Lesions are homogeneous and continuous.
- Crypt abscesses.
- Reduction in goblet cells.[186,193]

Common features

- Onset is usually in young adulthood, but it can develop at any age.
- The course of these diseases is characterised by flare-ups.
- Is accompanied by extra-digestive manifestations (joints, skin/mucous membranes, eyes).
- Carries a markedly heightened risk of colorectal cancer.
- Much more common in industrialised countries.
- No longer a rare disease.
- Less common in countries with poor hygiene.[190,193,194]

Application of endobiogenic medicine in IBS and IBD

Spasm of the colon

When there is a spasm in the colon, there is congestion and hyperreactivity present. There is hyperreactivity of the autonomic nervous system, which occurs in order to increase the contact time between chyme and the wall of the colon, therefore facilitating the absorption of a particular metabolite. Hence, when a spasm occurs, it is not simply by chance. There is a reason for it.[186]

Variation in stools

The appearance of the stools can help one distinguish problems originating in:

a) The small intestine and right colon if there are
   • copious stools, in the form of a frothy or fatty purée, foul-smelling, yellowish in colour.
   • presence of undigested food; blood and mucus very rare.
   • pain in the periumbilical region and right iliac fossa with borborygmus.
b) Left colon, if there are:
   • few stools, dark colour, little smell.
   • urgent defecation with gas, often mucus and blood.
   • pain in the left iliac fossa, hypogastric or sacral region.[186]

Metabolic end-purpose of the receptors in the colon

Table 23. Please refer to Figure 18 in Chapter 12 for the location of the receptors in the bowel

Hormone receptor	Metabolic end-purpose
ACTH	Water and electrolyte absorption
FSH and LH	Protein metabolism: • adaptation concerning structure and reconstruction: • elements controlled by ACTH, FSH, then TRH-TSH are all ones that provide for structure
PRL-GH TSH alone (slightly) TRH-TSH	Glucose metabolism: • process of immediate adaptation, whose end-purpose is action • concerns the terminal colon (the zone where cancers are most common)
TSH	Lipid metabolism

As mentioned in Chapter 12, the presence of the hormonal receptors in the colon is significant. However, they do not indicate the level of hormone present, but, rather, they indicate the level of functionality of the receptors in that particular location.

These receptors permit the phenomena of adaptation; they provide the last opportunity for a given metabolite to be absorbed and assimilated into the system. This can only occur at a particular part of the colon where the given receptor is located. Each part of the colon allows the absorption of nutrients or residues in accordance with the needs of each endocrine fraction.[186]

Autonomic nervous system elements inducing IBS

1. Vagal hypertonia
   - acceleration of transit, but no spasms
2. Strong alphasympathetic
   - if there are spasms occurring
   - if diarrhoea, then constipation (atony)
3. Strong betasympathetic
   - defecation in the morning (discharge, then nothing)

It is important to consider the state of the pelvic region in terms of stasis and congestion. Pelvic congestion can participate in the disorder present, hence the need to use specific plants capable of decongesting the pelvic region.[186]

IBD

As discussed previously, the prevalence of this dynamic, programmed and repetitive endocrine demand, in a specific location of the bowel, has as its consequence a process of selection of the local saprophytic flora favouring those elements that supply the required metabolic activity. This continues, up until the point where the autoimmune activity is initiated in order to neutralise the micro-organisms in question.

This explains the official findings with regards to the pathogenesis of IBD:

- Anomalous immune response of the gut, with regards to the components of bacterial flora.
- Inhibition of mechanisms of apoptosis.
- Modification of T lymphocytes of lamina propria which are not destroyed by apoptosis, and bearing witness to the inflammation produced by cytoplasmic proteolytic enzymes.
- Apparent intolerance of own intestinal flora, by an immune response directed against it.
- The consequent increase in adaptative activity due to a chronically elevated alphasympathetic activity.[186]

Crohn's disease and ulcerative colitis

From an endobiogenic perspective, Crohn's and ulcerative colitis represent a dysfunction in the regulation of the digestive tract—permanent, fundamental and adaptive. The organism at a digestive level is struggling with regard to adaptive maintenance.

Location of the lesions

The location confirms that a functional disorder is the true cause of the illness.

CD and UC seem to have the same aetiology, but in reality, the nature of the imbalance responsible for the illness is different.[186]

Application of endobiogeny in CD

Significance of the various sections of the bowels

a. The terminal ileum and the ileocecal junction are sites of absorption of different metabolites and of various electrolytes required for local catabolic balance.
b. The lower part of the cecum, then the cecum as a whole, is the site of stagnation of material destined for possible recovery, to be used for structural maintenance.
c. The ascending colon is responsible for the retrieval of material which is essential for use in construction and for the metabolic events associated with it.

This explains why this region is rich primarily in ACTH receptors.

Endobiogenic features present in Crohn's disease

- FSH +++
- Initial thyroid insufficiency resulting in an increase in TSH +++
- Disturbance of glucose and lipid metabolism. This leads to an increase in liver drainage, resulting in the alteration of the ecology of the ileum
- Strong parasympathetic activity
- Pancreatic insufficiency +++
- Strong alphasympathetic reactivity
- Corticoadrenal activity strong, but insufficient to inhibit ACTH or to meet structuro-functional adaptation demand
- Fairly strong androgenic activity but oestrogens relatively greater than androgens
- Very weak parathyroid (Chvostek +)

ANS and endocrine elements inducing CD

In Crohn's disease, there is high parasympathetic activity with a constant state of alphasympathetic reactivity and low betasympathetic activity. Because beta is low, the system is not able to reset itself, and the dysfunction continues. The disturbance at the level of the autonomic nervous system participates in the 'spasmophilic' state present in CD. *'The spasmophilia necessitates permanent extra restructuring based on a permanent exaggerated activation of the gonadotropic axis'.*[186]

In most cases, there is a gonadic inefficiency, therefore, an inadequate oestrogenic response. As a result, there is an increase in FSH. This is exacerbated by a constant activation of horizontal auto-adaptation: there is an over solicitation of ACTH, causing an excessive demand on the thyroid axis in order to respond to the anabolism solicited by FSH. However, there exists a fundamental peripheral thyroid insufficiency, as well as an insufficiency of the exocrine pancreas.

This induces the mechanisms responsible for the inflammation and diarrhoea: the peripheral thyroid insufficiency induces a central thyroid overactivity (high TRH and TSH) with a conflict of energy choice within the thyrotropic axis (between TRH and TSH) and its direct consequences of a conflict of influence between endocrine and exocrine pancreas. This results in an acceleration of bile flow in order to compensate for the pancreatic insufficiency. All of which generates gut dysbiosis and hence ileoce-cal lesions. There also exists a state of hyperinsulinism which is a major determining factor of free radical activity and inflammation.[186]

With regards to the relevance of the various segments of the bowels

- Crohn's disease is characterised by skip lesions, and this is not a coincidence. From an endobiogenic perspective, this is highly relevant and related to the particular hormone receptors involved in the disorder, as shown in Figure 19.

Symptomatic manifestations present in CD

- Masculine muscular appearance contrasting with feminine features.
- Persistent Chvostek through hypoparathyroidism.
- Quite keen on sport, as needs physical demand to get him/herself moving.
- Flare-ups in tune with an increase in oestrogen/androgen ratio—when androgens are low relative to oestrogens, there is a higher catabolic to anabolic activity which plays a major role in Crohn's disease. In Crohn's disease, there is a net catabolic activity.[186]

Application of endobiogeny in UC

The rectum and rectosigmoid junction are the final sites of absorption of water, electrolytes and various urgently needed metabolites before evacuation. It is the last chance the organism has to recuperate what is needed. This explains why these areas are rich primarily in ACTH receptors.

Endobiogenic features present in ulcerative colitis

- Strong parasympathetic ++++
- Pancreatic insufficiency
- Strong alphasympathetic ++ (sometimes violent)
- Weak peripheral thyroid activity with high central thyroid activity
- Very weak parathyroid (Chvostek +)
- Weak cortico-adrenal activity and growth hormone
- Frequent allergic phenomena

ANS and endocrine elements inducing UC

In ulcerative colitis there is a constant state of high alphasympathetic activity, which is caused by a fundamental insufficiency of the adrenal cortex. There is also, a high central thyroid activity (TRH, TSH). This is amplified by a deficient growth hormone activity, which as a result causes an exocrine pancreatic insufficiency and an exacerbation of an already overactive parasympathetic state. Due to the excessively raised alphasympathetic state and the deficient adrenal cortex, there is a permanent over secretion of ACTH. As in the case of CD, there is a state of hyperinsulinism which drives the inflammatory process.[186]

Symptomatic manifestations UC

- Frequent allergic symptoms with inflammatory infiltration of mucosa of the colon.
- Intra-parietal vascularity.
- Ulceration through secondary infection.
- Intolerance to cow's-milk proteins, which increase the inflammatory process.
- Immune factors: anti-colon antibodies, thus the development of an autoimmune state.

Treatment aims

In CD, it is necessary to

1. Reduce parasympathetic and alphasympathetic activity
2. Support adrenals
3. Support pancreatic activity
4. Reduce excessive central thyroid axis solicitation
5. Assess gonadotropic axis activity and treat as needed
6. Treat dysbiosis
7. Never carry out biliary drainage, as the bile flow is already accelerated

In UC, it is necessary to

1. Reduce hyper ACTH
2. Moderate the very strong alphasympathetic reactivity, which is not as continuous as in Crohn's, but is extremely violent
3. Strongly stimulate the adrenal gland
4. Support pancreas
5. Support peripheral thyroid activity and reduce central thyroid activity
6. Treat dysbiosis[186]

Phytotherapy

Use plant medicines with the following actions:

- Anti-inflammatory (Chapter 14, Table 24)
- Digestive antispasmodic (Table 16, Chapter 13)
- Sphincter of Oddi antispasmodics (Table 7, Chapter 5)
- Alphasympatholytic (Table 2, Chapter 3)
- Parasympatholytic (Table 3, Chapter 3)
- Adrenal support (Table 4, Chapter 3; Table 10, Chapter 8)
- Anti-central hyperthyroid; decreasing TRH, TSH (Table 13, Chapter 10)
- Peripheral thyroid stimulant (Table 13, Chapter 10)
- Anti-gonadotropic (Table 12, Chapter 9)
- Anti-insulin (Table 14, Chapter 11)
- Bactericidal (Table 15, Chapter 13)

If diarrhoea is present use plants containing tannins (Table 21, Chapter 13) and if constipation is present use plants containing mucilage, e.g. *Althea officinalis* and *Malva sylvestris*. When using these plants for their mucilaginous properties always use them in aqueous form.

Materia medica

Table 24. Anti-inflammatory plants[25,198–211]

Plant	Form used	Part used
Curcuma longa	Tincture, capsule	Root
Ribes nigrum GM	Glycerine macerate D1 dilution—bud, Infusion—leaf	Bud, leaf
Glycyrrhiza glabra	Tincture, fluid extract, decoction	Root
Boswellia serrata	Capsule, essential oil	Resin
Hydrastis canadensis	Tincture, capsule, decoction	Root
Matricaria chamomilla	Fluid extract, tincture, essential oil, infusion, capsule	Flower

CHAPTER FIFTEEN

Functional biology

The functional biology, also known as the biology of functions, is a biological modelling program that evaluates the functional capabilities of the neuroendocrine system. It is a unique blood test that does not evaluate serum levels. Rather, it evaluates the activity of the hormones at a cellular and tissular level, providing over 150 markers.

Classical lab data is based on binary considerations:

- Disease vs non-disease
- Normal vs abnormal[195]

Classical blood tests which evaluate serum levels of hormones do not look at how the hormones are functioning in the body and do not consider the notion of relativity.

> Serum levels of hormones reflect neither the degree of stimulation needed nor the metabolic costs incurred in producing a particular hormone.[195]

This is why, in many cases, a patient may be symtomatic but have normal blood test results. There are times when conventional hormone tests which look at serum levels will be normal, but if the time is taken to perform a thorough case history and examination one can find signs of a disorder.[195]

What do we conclude from this? Do we conclude:

a. That the patient is healthy, and no treatment is needed?
b. That the patient is somehow manifesting the symptoms due to a psychological problem and that they require psychiatric treatment?
c. That there is indeed a problem as the case history and examination findings prove and that maybe the standard blood tests are missing something?

The functional biology, helps the practitioner understand the aetiology of the dysfunctions at hand and in so doing devise an effective treatment plan. Rather than simply relying on patient symptoms, the functional biology allows the practitioner to evaluate the patients progress, numerically, over time.

Understanding the functional biology markers

We will now look at some of the important functional biology markers (indexes). We will not discuss all the indexes and will simply focus on the most relevant ones that are of most value within the scope of this book, and to the cases we will discuss later on.

Please remember that these results are very different to standard hormone tests where serum levels are evaluated. The functional biology does not looking at serum levels. It evaluates the effect of the hormones at a cellular and tissular level as well as the relative activity between one hormone and another. What is presented below, are how the indexes appear in the functional biology.

The relevant index appears on the left, then you will see a value for S and a value for F. The S value stands for Structure, and this is how the patient is functioning when in structure within that particular index. F stands for Function, and this is how the patient is in function, when active, within that particular index. Some patients have the ability to improve tremendously when active and are a lot worse in structure (when they are inside themselves, inside their mind). Likewise, some patients are better in structure than function and some similar in structure and function. The colour signifies whether the value is below normal, normal or above normal. Grey is low, white is normal, and black is high.

You will also see a number next to the colour so that you know the exact level of that particular index. To the far right, you will see the normal range for the index. You will now see the indexes with an explanation below them explaining what each index means.

Beta MSH/alpha MSH	s	● 1.58		6–8	☐
	f	○	1.58		☐

Beta MSH/alpha MSH: measures the relative activity of the betasympathetic verses the alphasympathetic.

| ACTH | s | ◐ 1e-3 | 0.71–3 | ☐ |
| | f | ◐ | 5e-4 | ☐ |

ACTH: measures the activity of the ACTH pituitary hormone. If low, it means that it is being suppressed by cortisol. If high, it means that there is enough pituitary stimulation to meet the demands of the organism in terms of adrenal stimulation.

When you see a value such as 1e–3, it means there are three zeros after the number, and because it is blue it is low, so in the minus. This value is –1000 so very low, but remember its low relative to cortisol not in the blood. We are not talking about serum levels of ACTH. This is very important to remember.

| Cortisol | s | ● 42.12 | 3–7 | ☐ |
| | f | ● | 32.96 | ☐ |

Cortisol: measures the activity of cortisol, which is the response of the adrenal gland in managing adaptation. When this index is elevated, it represents the level of mal-adaptive cortisol.

| Permissivity | s | ◐ 0.25 | 0.45–0.8 | ☐ |
| | f | ◐ | 0.20 | ☐ |

Permissivity: measures the activity of the adrenal gland in the synthesis and the secretion activity of other hormones (permissivity). Permissive cortisol is the positive effect of cortisol, i.e. its ability to facilitate the functioning of other endocrine organs.

This index allows one to understand the amount of adaptation effort needed by the adrenal gland:

• The less permissive the adrenal gland, the more the endocrine system works on stand-by mode, hence there is a reduction in the overall metabolism.
• A reduction in permissivity, due to a strong stress-based cortisol, can, however, be a factor of thyroid reactivation to increase the catabolism and restore overall metabolism.[196]

| Adrenal gland activity | s | ● 10.58 | 2.7–3.3 | ☐ |
| | f | ● | 6.48 | ☐ |

Adrenal gland activity: measures the global activity of the adrenal gland. It indicates whether the adrenal gland is weak or strong. It does not indicate whether it fulfils its duel role of adaptation and permissivity. In order to calculate this; you need the cortisol/adrenal gland ratio, so divide cortisol by adrenal gland activity. This should be around 3.

- A Ratio >3: means that cortisol is over-stimulated by ACTH. It means that there is a strong demand and response and either insufficiency of the adrenal gland or cortisol essentially adaptive with a limited permissive role.
- A Ratio <3: this means that the adrenal gland response is adequate.
- A Ratio <1: this is an extreme situation, there is a strong adrenal gland activity and weak cortisol, permissivity dominates, and adaptation becomes purely permissive (adaptation-permissivity < 0).[196]

| Peripheral serotonin | s | ● 37.76 | | 1.5–7.5 | ☐ |
| | f | ● | 29.55 | | ☐ |

Peripheral serotonin: is an inverse marker. It measures the level of activity of peripheral serotonin. By extension, it gives some indication of the level of central serotonin. Remember that serotonin stimulates parasympathetic activity.

| Histamine activity | s | ◐ 0.93 | | 20–60 | ☐ |
| | f | ◐ | 1.53 | | ☐ |

Histamine activity: measures the activity of circulating histamine. Remember that histamine is linked to alphasympathetic activity and that it prolongs the life of alpha and retards the activity of beta.

- Usually, low histamine implies a strong adrenal gland and the adaptation is well managed.
- Conversely, a high histamine implies a weak adrenal gland.

However, it may be the case that histamine is high in spite of a normal adrenal gland activity; this may occur when the adaptation demand is weak (high adaptation index) or when the cortisol response is insufficient (high eosinophilia). Histamine is put into action when there is chronic stress in order to retard the activity of Beta, as histamine is the autacoid of alpha.[196]

| Potential histamine | s | ◐ 1.97 | | 6–12 | ☐ |
| | f | ◐ | 3.63 | | ☐ |

Potential histamine: measures the number of histamine receptors ready for use. It shows how the person internalises stress.

| Inflammation | s | ◐ 0.05 | | 0.3–2.5 | ☐ |
| | f | ◐ | 0.07 | | ☐ |

Inflammation: measures internal inflammatory activity.

Insulin	s	● 5.45		1.5–5	☐
	f	○	4.27		☐

Insulin: measures the level of the endocrino-metabolic activity of insulin.

Insulinic resistance	s	◔ 0.04		0.75–1.25	☐
	f	○	0.06		☐

Insulinic resistance: measures the level of inhibition of the membrane activity of insulin, independently of its temporary activity, linked to adaptation. Insulin resistance will increase in times of stress to prevent glucose from entering the cells. This is in order to ensure that the priority organs (heart, brain, muscles …) get enough energy.

Splanchnic congestion	s	● 51.05		0.011–0.163	
	f	●	10.07		☐

Splanchnic congestion: measures the relative level of active congestion in the splanchnic reservoir. The splanchnic region is one of the major centres of congestion in the organism. Splanchnic congestion increases in times of adaptation. This is to allow the particular organ or group of organs under stress, greater nutrition and oxygenation.[196]

Progesterone	s	● 97.39		3–6	☐
	f	●	54.67		☐

Progesterone: measures the activity of the progesterone.

FSH	s	◔ 0.02		0.57–8	☐
	f	○	0.01		☐

FSH: measures the activity of the pituitary follicle-stimulating hormone.

LH	s	◔ 4e-3		0.34–4	☐
	f	○	2e-3		☐

LH: measures the activity of the pituitary luteinising hormone.

Genital ratio	s	◔ 0.32		0.8–0.95	☐
	f	○	0.32		☐

Genital ratio: measures the ratio of the global activity of androgens versus oestrogens.

Genital androgens	s	◔ 0.07		0.18–0.22	☐
	f	◔	0.12		☐

Genital androgens: measures the level of metabolic activity of the genital androgens.

| Genital oestrogens | s | ● 0.17 | | 0.1–0.14 | ☐ |
| | f | ● | 0.28 | | ☐ |

Genital oestrogens: measures the level of metabolic activity of the genital oestrogens.

| Folliculin | s | ◐ 0.10 | | 0.9–1.5 | ☐ |
| | f | ◯ | 0.17 | | ☐ |

Folliculin: measures the oestrogenic activity in its folliculin sourcing.

| Peripheral oestrogens | s | ● 2.1e5 | | 100–2300 | ☐ |
| | f | ● | 7.1e5 | | ☐ |

Peripheral oestrogens: measures the organo-tissular global activity of peripheral oestrogens, relative to the FSH stimulation.

| Cata-ana ratio | s | ● 3.82 | | 1.8–3 | ☐ |
| | f | ● | 5.45 | | ☐ |

Cata/ana ratio: measures the relationship between catabolism and anabolism, and it is an indicator of the installation of the general adaptation syndrome against the aggression.

| Bone remodeling | s | ◯ 7.80 | | 2.5–8.5 | ☐ |
| | f | ◯ | 7.80 | | ☐ |

Bone remodelling: measures the bone remodelling activity and the extent of bone impairment.

| Thyroid metabolic | s | ● 15.66 | | 3.5–5.5 | ☐ |
| | f | ● | 15.66 | | ☐ |

Thyroid metabolic: measures the metabolic activity of the thyroid.

Definitions taken from Endobiogenic Medical Assistant 3.0 (algorithm-based software used to generate the functional biology indexes from the base data).

CHAPTER SIXTEEN

Endobiogenic physical examination

W e will now look at some of the endobiogenic physical examination techniques. This is not an exhaustive list of examination techniques, and we will only cover what is most relevant.

The physical examination must certainly never be undervalued or skipped, as it provides a vast amount of information that would otherwise have been overlooked. It is essential that the practitioner takes the time to perform an in-depth physical examination.

Findings relative to the autonomic nervous system

Parasympathetic

Examination signs and symptoms linked to a high parasympathetic state.

- Overweight as para is an anabolic state. This is not always the case as it depends on other catabolic and anabolic factors present in the organism.
- Slumped posture.
- Walking slowly.
- Introverted, shy, quiet.
- Damp/sweaty hands.
- Excessive salivation.
- Enlarged parotids.
- Increased gut motility/diarrhoea.
- Tired after eating a meal.
- Signs of splanchnic congestion, e.g. over pancreatic and liver regions.

- Concave chest.
- Recurrent infections, e.g. enlarged and infected tonsils, recurrent cystitis etc.
- Nausea.
- Frequent urge to pass urine, especially at night.

Alphasympathetic

Examination signs and symptoms linked to a high alphasympathetic state.

- Fast blink response (startle response).
- Slim as alpha is a catabolic system. This is not always the case as it depends on other catabolic and anabolic factors present in the organism.
- Cold hands and or cold feet.
- Very ticklish. Alpha increases the sensitivity of the patient.
- Redness in the face as alpha constricts the capillaries and the blood pools in the skin.
- Red freckles on the skin. Caused by very high alpha in a specific location at a particular time. Alpha is constrictive and causes the blood to pool in that region.
- Fast reflexes.
- Jumpy/fidgety.
- Congestion, e.g. splanchnic congestion, adrenal congestion as alpha participates in the phenomenon of congestion due to its constriction.
- Hypertension.

Betasympathetic

Examination signs and symptoms that are linked to a low betasympathetic state (insufficient adrenal activity).

- Inability to cope with stress.
- Fatigue.
- Allergic states as cortisol has an antihistamine activity.
- Cold hands and feet as beta has a dilatory effect on blood vessels. In this case, there is a high alpha and deficient beta.
- Congestion maintained as beta is the release mechanism.
- Congestion upon rolling over the adrenal region.

Examination signs and symptoms that are linked to a high peripheral betasympathetic state (overactive adrenals) and high central betasympathetic (elevated TRH).

- Explosive personality. Quick to anger as beta is the release mechanism. TRH is also implicated here as TRH is central beta.
- High Central beta (TRH), anxiety states, obsessiveness, quick thinker, always planning ahead, can be a creative personality, very active mind. Vivid dreams and dreams in colour.

- Strong handshake, firm.
- Walks with energy, brisk walker.
- Loud voice.
- Warm hands.
- Strong urine flow implies a good beta.
- Low histamine or blocked histamine expression.
- Possibility of palpitations.

Observation

It is important to note that the examination of the patients starts as soon as you first lay eyes on the patient. A vast amount of information can be obtained from observation.
   Observe the patient as they walk towards your clinic room:

- What is there posture like?
- How do they walk?

Is their chest open and do they stand up very straight? Are they hunched over? Do they walk briskly and move with energy and intension? Do they walk very slowly?
   Be mindful of the following:

- What is their handshake like? Is it limp, or do they grip your hand firmly and squeeze hard?
- How do they speak? Do they talk softly and quietly? Do they sit in the consultation quietly, and is it hard to extract the information from them? Are they loud? Do they constantly talk, so much so that you cannot say much in the consultation? Are they sitting still or do they constantly fidgety.
- What is there complexion like?
- What is their body shape like, and how is the fat distributed?

From the very beginning, from when you first meet the patient, if you pay attention, you can discern valuable information about the patient. You will start to understand how the autonomic nervous system and the endocrine system is functioning in that patient. You will start to get an idea of the patient's terrain.

Examination

Hands and feet

- Are the hands and feet cold? If they are cold, it implies that there is high alphasym-pathetic activity. This is because alpha is a constrictive system and as such con-stricts the blood vessels and impedes circulation.

Some patients say to me, 'Yes my hands are cold, but it is cold outside'. It may be cold outside, but they have been inside the clinic for an hour or so, so their body has time to adapt. When you examine several patients in this way and become aware of this finding, you can see that you may have a patient attend your clinic at the peak of summer and their hands can be freezing cold. You may see a patient in the winter, and their hands may be warm.

If you are stressed, you may realise that your hands are very cold. If you sit still and perform a meditative exercise for say 15 minutes and if you manage to relax, you will notice your hands become warm. This is because you are successfully rebalancing your autonomic nervous system and reducing your alphasympathetic activity.

- Are the feet colder than the hands? If this is the case, it is due to pelvic congestion. When the pelvic area is congested, the blood flow to the feet is impaired, and the feet will be colder than the hands. The hands may also be cold, but it is the temperature difference we are looking for. Pelvic congestion will be present in conditions like cystitis, fibroids and benign prostate hypertrophy.
- Are the hands and feet damp and sweaty? If they are it is because the parasympathetic nervous system is overactive.

Eyes

- Ask the patient to close their eyes gently; look at their eyelids. Do they tremble? If so, it a sign of high TRH (high central beta activity).
- Glabellar tap. When the patient is lying down on the examination couch: tap your finger a few times on the glabella quickly without warning the patient. If the startle response/blink response is exaggerated, this is linked to a high alphasympathetic state. It is important that the patient is not expecting it, though, as it will diminish their response and not give you a true indication.
- At this point, you may wish to check the reflexes, as brisk reflexes are also a sign of high TRH.
- Look at the pupil size:
  - Miosis (excessive constriction of the pupil)—high para
  - Mydriasis (dilation of the pupil)—high alpha

Tongue

- Look at the tongue:
  - A flat white tongue means colon congestion and dysbiosis

Lymph nodes

- Palpate the parotid glands. If they are enlarged, it means that there is exocrine pancreatic insufficiency and high parasympathetic activity. The parotids will enlarge if the exocrine pancreas is insufficient as they try to compensate for impaired digestion. In addition to this, palpate the other lymph nodes in the region.

Torso

- Examine the chest. If the central region of the chest is concave, it is linked to high parasympathetic activity in structure. See Figure 20. The parasympathetic system is responsible for inverting and internalising. On an emotional level, patients with a very high para can internalise and not express themselves.

Rolling the skin

If the organ underneath is congested, e.g. pancreas, liver, gallbladder (splanchnic region), then the skin is pulled down tight over the organ. When you roll the skin, the skin will be tight, hard to lift and roll. It will be painful for the patient. This reflects signs of congestion.

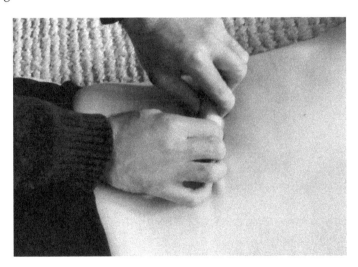

Figure 20. Rolling the skin.

Rolling is performed

- Over the liver and pancreatic region, starting from the side to the solar plexus—if there is tenderness and tightness, there is congestion.
- Up and down the back. If there is tightness and pain over the adrenal region, it is a sign of adrenal congestion. When rolling the skin also check to see if there is excessive redness as this is a sign of excessive histamine activity.

Abdomen

When palpating the abdomen, there are specific points in relation to endobiogenic medicine, that must be considered. As discussed in Chapter 12, there are various receptors in specific locations of the large intestine. Tenderness in these points will provide information as to which hormones are implicated in the condition.

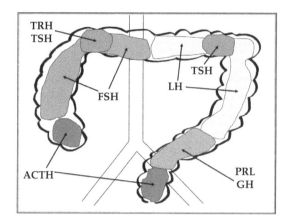

Figure 19. From Chapter 12.

FSH/LH involvement

- FSH/LH—press firmly over each eyebrow with your thumb and push away from the centre following the eyebrow. Check to see which side is more painful. The right means more FSH activity and the left means more LH activity.

Oestrogen

Signs of high oestrogenic activity:

- Long eyelashes. Conversely, short eyelashes mean weak oestrogen activity.
- Hyperlaxity of the joints.
- Fat deposits on the hips and curvy hips.
- Large breasts.
- Smooth skin.

Androgens

Signs of high androgenic activity:

- Broad shoulders.
- Good musculature.
- Excessive hair on the body.
- Black hair more in favour of androgens.

Prolactin

Signs of high prolactin activity:

- Large curve on the dorsal aspect of the foot.
- Large breasts.
- Pale milky skin.

Cortisol

Signs of high cortisol activity:

- Fat on the nape of the neck.
- Fat around the abdomen.
- Fat deposits at the back of the upper arm.

Insulin

Signs of high insulin:

- Fat deposits around the abdomen.

Reference: Information on Endobiogenic examination techniques obtained from observation in Dr Lapraz's clinic and seminar training programmes.

CHAPTER SEVENTEEN

Green clay

Green clay is truly a fantastic medicine and an indispensable tool in any natural pharmacy. I never travel without it. I use it extensively in my clinic, for both internal and external ailments. For the treatment of Crohn's and ulcerative colitis, it is highly effective for healing the gastrointestinal mucosa. The only time I would not use it would be if there was a stricture of the bowel. In this case, it may be possible to use the clay water and not to consume the clay sediment. This would depend on the case at hand.

A surgeon who attended my clinic, testified to a miraculous cure that she had witnessed first-hand in Africa by a local healer using green clay and plant medicines mixed together. The patient had developed gangrene on their foot and this surgeon had said that conventionally they would have had to amputate the foot. She was absolutely stunned by the cure she had witnessed.

Historical use of clay

The practice of geophagy, which involves the consumption of clay from the earth, is an ancient practice. It was performed by both humans and animals in order to

1. Elicit a healing effect on the gastrointestinal mucosa
2. Detoxify the body
3. Replenish mineral stores[197]

Clays have been employed for both internal and external afflictions and have highly absorptive and adsorptive properties. Adsorption is the adhesion of molecules or particles to a solid surface. It is these properties that make clay so effective at removing toxins from the body. Traditionally, clay minerals are mixed with water for various periods of time before use.[212]

Antibacterial effects of French green clay

Microbiological testing of French green clay, demonstrates its effectiveness at killing a broad spectrum of human pathogens. However, not all clays are antibacterial. Many clays have healing effects on the tissues of the body due to their adsorptive properties, but this does not make them antibacterial.[213]

In a study designed to evaluate the antibacterial effects of French green clay, two types of clay (CsAg02 and CsAr02) were tested against a number of gram-negative, gram-positive and mycobacterial pathogens. Only CsAg02 demonstrated antibacterial activity. It exhibited

> an extraordinary ability to kill pathogenic E. coli, Salmonella enterica serovar Typhimurium, P. aeruginosa, ESBL E. coli (which is resistant to 11 antibiotics), and Mycobacterium marinum (a species genetically closely related to M. ulcerans) as well as inhibit the growth of pathogenic S. aureus, penicillin-resistant S. aureus (PRSA), methicillin-resistant S. aureus (MRSA; and also resistant to 10 antibiotics).

The exact mechanism of action of how clay is able to kill these pathogens is not fully understood yet.[213]

Endobiogenic use of green clay

From the early 1970s, Drs Duraffourd and Lapraz observed that many of their patients were using green clay for a variety of disorders. This was intriguing and so prompted them to investigate the therapeutic role green clay could have in a clinical setting.

Dr Rozenn Dodeur, a doctor and anesthesiologist responsible for palliative care at the hospital of Châteadun, pioneered the use of green illite clay in combination with a variety of essential oils. This preparation is known as Escargil® and is a product that is used externally. Internally, green clay is simply mixed with water for a number of hours in order to activate it, before consumption.

Formulation of Escargil®:

- Green illite clay
- Aloe vera
- Essential oils of *Lavandula angustifolia*, *Eugenia caryophyllata* and *Rosmarinus officinalis*

The essential oils and aloe vera in this preparation enhance the effect of the green clay. They have anti-inflammatory, antiseptic and circulatory stimulatory properties.[214]

The effect of Escargil® was remarkable. It was able to treat and cure:

- shingles
- numerous eschars (necrotic tissue from burns or gangrene)
- leg ulcers
- various wounds and sores, especially of diabetic origin
- rheumatic pain

What was fascinating, was that the putrid odour associated with the eschars would disappear within 24 to 48 hours of applying the Escargil®.[214]

Properties of green clay

Internally:

- Anti-inflammatory
- Vulnerary and anti-haemorrhagic
- Anti-infectious
- Anti-fungal
- Anthelminthic
- Antidiarrheal
- Adsorbent and demulcent
- Absorbent

Internally: Green clay is highly effective in the treatment of gastrointestinal disorders. These include, peptic and duodenal ulceration, gastritis, enteritis, Crohn's, ulcerative colitis, diarrhoea, fungal and parasitic infections. Drs Duraford and Lapraz used French green clay internally with great success in the treatment of cholera.

Externally:

- Purifying
- Anti-inflammatory
- Antiseptic
- Anti-fungal
- Healing
- Anti-oedema
- *'Modifier of nucleocytoplasmic relationship in vaginal cells'*[214]

Externally: Green clay has been shown to be effective in the treatment of burns, infected wounds, ulcers, abscesses, boils, acne, fungal infections, thrush and vaginitis.

Toxicity

In clinical trials, no toxicity has been discovered from the use of illite green clay. Furthermore, no increase in blood or urinary aluminium levels were detected.[214]

CHAPTER EIGHTEEN

What about the diet?

In my experience, when dealing with patients who present with digestive disorders, modification of the diet is an essential part of the treatment. The patients that really take this on board and follow the advice, will do the best. Generally, the more severe the condition, the more work the patient will need to put into their diet.

Food is addictive, and patients can make up all kinds of reasons, as to why they can't give up specific foods. I had a patient with Crohn's disease who said they needed to keep drinking Coca-Cola daily, as it was helping their Crohn's disease. Of course, it is not easy to change your diet, especially if you have been eating particular foods all of your life, and many of these foods are addictive. Patients can go through withdrawal. Sugar, dairy and gluten are all addictive.[215-219]

When a patient is giving up addictive foods, it is very important to support the nervous system and the adrenal glands with the use of supplements and plant medicines. Withdrawal from these addictive substances is an aggression on the organism. The stress induced will affect the corticotropic axis.

Some time ago, a patient with Crohn's disease came to see me at my clinic. They saw a great benefit in a very short time from the treatment and dietary changes. So much so that their symptoms had improved by about 70 to 80%. When they came back for the follow-up appointment, they expressed how much better they were and they had realised how the diet had helped them. However, they said that they would not carry on with the treatment, as they could not follow the diet anymore. They were not willing to stop eating refined carbohydrates, sugar, junk foods etc. This was a great shame, as many of us know what can happen in Crohn's disease if it is not managed in the right way. In a way that actually addresses the underlying mechanisms and actually promotes deep healing to the gut.

Dietary modification is not the sole treatment modality used in IBD and we have discussed the mechanisms involved earlier on in this book; but the dietary aspect is not to be missed, as it can make all the difference as to whether treatment will be successful. In fact, more and more research is coming to light, proving that none of us should be following this so-called modern diet that we have adopted.

Modifying diet in children

I find in my clinic that the reality is that children adapt much easier to dietary change, as they are more flexible psychologically. Their organism adapts much easier as a whole. Adults are more ridged and are not so ready to change their ways. It is really the parents that have issues, with regards to changing their child's diet. They worry about how their child will feel if they stop giving them sweets and chocolates. They feel guilty if they do not give these foods to their children. There is this notion that this is what children eat: sweets and chocolates. Parents feel that they are bad parents if they do not give these foods to their children and often worry about what others will think. So, parents are feeling guilty for the wrong reasons. Guilty if they do not give their children inflammatory foods, foods that promote disease, instead of foods that promote health. We are not talking about the odd treat here. We are talking about consuming these unhealthy snacks on a daily basis, combined with poor meal choices. This has disastrous effects on the body.

What sort of diet is best for healing the gut, body and mind?

Generally, we need to choose a diet which is anti-inflammatory and packed with nutrient-dense foods. A diet which promotes healing to the gut lining (epithelium). Once this occurs, the patient will start to absorb nutrients fully again, and positive change will occur.

Conventionally, nearly all consultants tell patients with IBD that there is no proof that diet will affect them and that they can eat what they like. In fact, I have heard directly from consultants and from patients who have been advised by their consultants that they should consume a lot of ice cream and cake in order to put weight on.

In my clinic, I tend to use three types of diets for my patients:

1. Sugar, gluten, dairy and caffeine-free
2. Paleo diet
3. GAPS diet

If patients are strict vegan or vegetarian, then I modify the diet in the best way possible.

1. The sugar-free, gluten-free, dairy-free, caffeine-free diet
The aim of this diet, is to follow a low-carb and refined carb-free diet. It is important to consume plenty of vegetables, and the patient should have a moderate amount

of good fats. This diet is aimed at stabilising blood glucose and reducing inflammation. Removing all preservatives, artificial colourings, flavourings, and sweeteners is essential. It is a clean wholesome diet. Home cooking is a must with the use of fresh ingredients. Organic foods should be ideally consumed if possible. This is to avoid pesticide, hormones and other toxic substances. The diet listed below often needs to be modified for specific patients. For example, if you are dealing with a patient with IBS who has diarrhoea, it would be a good idea to avoid the grains with high fibre content such as quinoa and brown rice, as they are likely to irritate the intestines.

These are the foods allowed:

Carbohydrates: small amounts of the following complex carbohydrates are allowed: sweet potato, brown rice, quinoa and buckwheat. Pumpkin and butternut squash are also permitted.

Protein: pork, chicken, lamb, beef, duck, guinea fowl, fish, eggs etc. Make sure it is organic or free-range. Make sure it is free from hormones and antibiotics. Fish should be wild-caught and not from a farm due to the hormones used. Avoid tuna and swordfish due to high levels of mercury.

Fats: avocado, unsalted raw nuts and seeds (these can also be activated for better absorption). Nut butters without added sugar. Coconut, olive, hemp, flax, pumpkin seed oils. They should be cold-pressed.

Milk alternatives: pure unsweetened coconut milk and unsweetened almond milk.

Organic vegetables and salads: good size portions for lunch and dinner. Vegetables can also be eaten for breakfast. It is better to have vegetables instead of salads for dinner for those who have fermentation issues.

Fermented foods: these are good for immunity and bowel health. Beet kvass, raw sauerkraut, kefir, tempeh, miso (only from health food shops not from restaurants as miso often contains MSG). Make sure these are raw and from a good brand.

Juicing: Juicing is very good but should be mainly vegetable juice. Only a small amount of fruit should be used for flavour. For those who have hypothyroidism, it is not recommended to juice Brassica family vegetables. Juicing should not be used in the early treatment of patients presenting with diarrhoea.

Mushrooms: these are especially good for immunity. Shiitake, maitake and reishi.

Example diet

Breakfast: eggs (boiled, scrambled, omelette with mushrooms and veg), avocado, smoked salmon or Parma ham (no sugar added), coconut yoghurt, chia seed pudding made with coconut milk or coconut yoghurt with nuts and cinnamon, nuts and seeds, paleo cereal made with nuts and seeds, paleo bread recipes made with; coconut flour, ground almonds, flax seeds etc.

Porridge: small amounts of quinoa porridge with lots of nuts and seeds and possibly desiccated coconut without sulphates. Again, this depends on the amount of fibre permitted.

Never have fruit for breakfast. Fruit should only be eaten between meals and eaten with nuts or nut butter.

Snacks: nut butter with fruit and coconut oil, plain nuts, coconut, almond, or cashew yoghurt, hummus (depending on the patient) with carrot sticks, celery sticks with nut butter, homemade energy balls.

Lunch: half a plate of salad or vegetables with a dressing made of one of the good oils listed above, lemon and apple cider vinegar. Small amounts of the complex carbohydrates listed above, portion of protein from the list above, lentils are allowed on occasion.

Meat stock, as described in the GAPS diet section, is highly beneficial and should be consumed on a daily basis.

Dinner: same as lunch, ideally a smaller meal and at least 3 hours before bedtime. If fat loss is required, avoid all complex carbohydrates at dinner time or fast (skip dinner) or simply have a green juice.

Paleo diet

I will not go into this in detail as there is so much information already available on this diet. I use this diet for patients that require a grain-free diet as part of the treatment process.

GAPS diet

This is the diet that I prefer to use with all my autoimmune patients. I particularly like the stages in the GAPS diet, as it allows for much deeper healing to the epithelium of the bowel and can yield faster results. The stages are important; by introducing foods at different times, it allows patients to identify foods that are not tolerated. This diet works very well with IBD where there is a lot of inflammation, ulceration and damage to the gut lining.

The GAPS diet was developed by Dr Natasha Campbell McBride based on her many years of clinical experience. The GAPS diet is based on the specific carbohydrate diet (SCD) created by Dr Sidney Valentine Haas, in order to treat chronic inflammatory conditions in the digestive tract.

The SCD diet was made famous after a mother, Elaine Gottschall, healed her child of ulcerative colitis. Elaine went on to become the author of a book called *Breaking the Vicious Cycle: Intestinal Health Through Diet*.

Interview with Dr Natasha Campbell McBride

In my interview with Dr Campbell McBride, she states that there is now an epidemic of people with abnormal gut flora and that these abnormalities are getting worse with every generation. Humanity is heading for a crisis.

The GAPS nutritional protocol was designed in order to drive out pathogens from the digestive tract and to re-establish normal gut flora or more accurately said; individual normal gut flora, as each person is unique. The GAPS protocol is used to heal and seal the gut wall.

Abnormal gut flora damages the integrity of the gut wall, making it leaky and porous. Microbes can then enter the body through the damaged gut wall, effecting the organism. Furthermore, the pathogenic gut flora, which feeds off the food in the gut, produce very toxic chemicals which exacerbate the condition.

When there is a leaky gut, partially undigested food absorbs into the system creating immune reactions. Food allergies and intolerances occur. If this process goes on for long enough, it can lead to autoimmune disease. The GAPS protocol assists in rebuilding the gut wall of the patient. In order to produce health epithelial cells to rebuild the gut wall, vast amounts of nutrients are required, and the GAPS diet provides ample amounts of these building materials. The GAPS diet reduces inflammation and assists in dampening down the autoimmune response, thus allowing healthy epithelial cells to develop unimpeded and regeneration of the lining of the bowel can occur.[220]

Autoimmunity form a GAPS perspective

Dr Campbell McBride believes that all autoimmunity is born in the gut. *'Our digestive system is the biggest immune organ in our body'*. The gut flora is a major source of data and provides valuable information for the immune system to act upon.

Dr Campbell McBride believes one of the major mechanisms of autoimmunity is toxicity. Specific toxins that are absorbed have an affinity for certain proteins in the body. These toxins attach themselves to the proteins and change their three-dimensional structure. One-third of all protein in the body is collagen and collagen contains large quantities of sulphur-containing amino acids. The primary role of sulphur in the body is detoxification. As collagen contains so much sulphur, it gets contaminated first, as the sulphur latches onto these toxins. The immune system then discovers these modified proteins and attacks them, thinking that they are invaders. As so much of the body is made up of collagen, the immune system attacks the very structure of the body. Usually, the body would use a nonspecific cell-mediated response or complement cascade, etc. In this case, an inflammatory reaction will occur in that part of the body where there is contaminated protein. As the inflammation becomes chronic due to toxicity, the immune system starts to develop antibodies against this tissue.

Dr Campbell McBride says, that in order to treat any autoimmune disease, no matter how far away from the gut it seems, you need to start from the gut, i.e. treat the digestive system (intestine). Even if patients do not present with specific digestive problems, you still need to start treating the gut. Dr Campbell McBride goes on to say, 'these particular patients are harder to convince', they can't see the connection with the gut as they have no obvious digestive issues. Specific tests for gut flora and leaky gut can be used to provide evidence of intestinal disturbance. In Dr Campbell

McBride's experience, the GAPS protocol has helped tens of thousands of individuals with autoimmune disease.

In Dr Campbell McBride's opinion, patients with severe autoimmune disease should follow the GAPS diet for the rest of their lives. In mild conditions, patients can follow the diet for approximately 2 years. The GAPS diet can fulfil all the nutritional needs. GAPS is a very nourishing and nutrient-dense diet. It removes nutritional deficiencies rapidly. It will rebalance the immune system and allow it to function optimally. Many patients can introduce grains again after the gut has been healed and are fine with them. It really depends on the patient.[220]

The microbiome

The gut microbiota lives deep within the gut wall, deep in the mucosa; it lives in harmony with the rest of the body. As mentioned earlier, toxins disrupt the finely balanced ecosystem of the bowel. The world is full of man-made toxic chemicals, and when these toxins effect the microbiome of a mother, the dysbiotic flora is then passed onto the infant during the birthing process via the birthing canal. Toxins can also have a more direct effect on the foetus. By the time a woman falls pregnant, her toxic load could be very high, and unfortunately, pregnancy is a way of the body ridding itself of these toxins. It offloads the toxins into the foetus.

According to Dr Campbell McBride, food has a far more powerful effect on the microbiome of the gut than probiotics do, and that's why the GAPS diet is so effective at dealing with dysbiosis. Dr Campbell McBride believes that none of us can digest gluten. Even if people are not experiencing obvious symptoms, the gluten is irritating the lining of the bowel.

Basis of the GAPS diet

Dr Campbell McBride looked at the research carried out by Dr Weston A. Price and also examined closely the basic nature and function of the human digestive system. As a result, she came to the conclusion that meat, fish, eggs and dairy (in the GAPS protocol only certain forms of dairy are used) are the only foods that the human digestive system can easily digest and assimilate into its own structure. Indeed, the protein composition in the human organism is very similar to the proteins found in these foods. In relation to human fat, when we analyse the composition in its biochemical structure, it is very similar to the fat found in meat, fish, eggs and dairy. The majority of the fats found in the body are saturated fats, and the second biggest group is monounsaturated. The body is constantly rebuilding and renewing itself, and it needs the correct building materials to do so. The best building material is animal-based fats and proteins. When plant material is analysed in the laboratory, we find that their amino acid composition is wrong for building human proteins. Some amino acids are in excess, and some are lacking. This is also the case with regards to plant-based fats. There are far too many polyunsaturated and monounsaturated fats. The biggest problem, however, is that they are indigestible to the human digestive system. The human stomach cannot digest plants.

So, what are plants for? Plants are the cleansers; they are there to cleanse the body and provide a valuable source of fibre. Plants also provide some vitamins, minerals and enzymes but not much of the proteins and fats required, as our digestive system can't adequately digest and absorb them. The large intestine which is at the end of the digestive tract and contains most of the flora will assist in some of the digestion of the plant material, but not much absorption will occur. Most of the absorption occurs higher up in the digestive system. The main purpose of plant matter/fibre is to feed the intestinal flora in the colon. Here, some of the sugars are converted into fatty acids. Butyrate, a short-chain fatty acid is very important for health, and as discussed earlier, there is a link between low levels of butyrate and Crohn's disease. Animal foods feed the body, and the plant foods cleanse the body.

Fifty per cent of the dry weight of the human body is fat; fat is a structural part of the body and extremely import. As Dr Campbell McBride says, 'eating fats is not optional' it is necessary and vital. The bulk of fat consumption has to come from animal fats. This is based on Dr Campbell McBride's research, and her views are based on her extensive clinical experience and the experience of other holistic doctors.[220]

GAPS diet stages

The GAPS diet consists of several stages, and working through each stage provides the best healing for the digestive system. However, Dr Campbell McBride says that if it is very difficult for patients to follow each stage of the GAPS protocol, they can simply start on the full GAPS diet. What is essential, though, is the GAPS soup (meat stock-based soup), and this must be a daily affair for GAPS people. When using pork, it is best to marinate it in raw sauerkraut or other fermented vegetables, as the enzymes and microbes in the fermented vegetables begin to predigest the meat.

The most therapeutic parts of the animal are the gelatinous parts. They are the most nutritious. These are the parts around the joints, neck, bones, head, the skin, tail and feet. Organ meats are very nutritious as well. It is not advisable to eat the lean muscle of the animal. You need the fatty, gelatinous parts.[220] In fact, I have read that hunter-gather tribes would keep the most prized cuts, which were the fatty cuts for themselves and would give the lean meat to the dogs.

Manual therapy in the treatment of abdominal adhesions

A bdominal adhesions can occur due to radiotherapy and inflammatory activity but are largely associated with surgery. Studies show that up to 90% of patients that undergo abdominal surgery developed abdominal adhesions. The extent of the adhesive disorder is dependent on the complexity of the initial surgical procedure.[221, 222]

Abdominal adhesions: what are they?

Abdominal adhesions are bands of fibrous tissue that can form between abdominal tissues and organs. Normally, the internal tissues and organs should slide freely amongst themselves as the body moves. They should not be stuck together. When abdominal adhesions are present, they cause tissues and organs in the abdominal cavity to adhere to one another; impeding movement and thus causing restrictions.[223]

Abdominal adhesions are known to cause partial or total small bowel obstructions. When this occurs, the intestinal contents cannot pass through the intestine. Patients may present with the following signs and symptoms; abdominal spasm with severe pain, loss of appetite, nausea, vomiting and distension.[222, 223]

Small bowel obstructions can become life-threatening and may require immediate surgery. In some cases, the surgeon may simply be able to lyse the adhesions, but if this is not possible a bowel resection will be required. There are many risks with this type of surgery, and these include, infection, bowel rupture and of course the development of more adhesions due to the surgical procedure.[223]

To date, there is no effective treatment available within the conventional medical model for abdominal adhesions. Indeed, all of the surgeons that I have spoken to say the same thing, that unless the adhesions are life-threatening, i.e. have caused complete bowel obstruction that does not resolve or caused strangulation of the bowel, they do not advise further surgery. This is because surgery causes adhesions. It is possible that the patient could end up worse than they were and lose more and more segments of bowel with each operation. Therefore, if patients present with obstructions, the preferred treatment from a classical medical perspective is to provide bowel rest and pain management and to wait to see if the obstruction resolves. The patient will not consume any foods or liquids for a period of time and will be placed on a drip to keep them hydrated. Analgesic and antispasmodic medications are administered and, in some cases, a nasogastric tube is inserted. If the patient is not in severe pain, then they may get away with simply staying on clear liquids for a period of time until the pain subsides.

These obstructions affect patients to varying degrees, and I have seen a whole variety in my clinic; ranging from a one-off attack to periodic severe episodes of pain and vomiting which can occur several times per year.

Some patients will present with constant generalised pain and tenderness on palpation in the abdominal area at and around the site of surgery and where the anastomosis is.

ADHESIONS

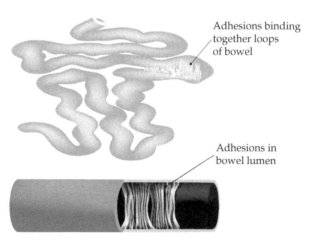

Figure 21. Adhesions of the bowel.

Is there another option for these patients?

According to experts in the field of manual therapy, and from what I have seen in my clinic, it would seem so. What follows is a series of interviews from three highly experienced therapists from the UK and USA who use hands-on work in order to treat patients with adhesion-related issues.

Some of these practitioners call themselves bodyworkers or hands-on therapists, but regardless of the name used they are employing a range of techniques; manually, in order to effect positive change in the fascia and viscera of the body. When dealing with patients suffering from abdominal adhesions, manual therapy is a very important aspect of treatment that should be used alongside the internal treatments that we prescribe in endobiogenic medicine.

I interviewed Amanda Oswald from the United Kingdom; Marty Ryan and Isabel Spradlin from the United States. Both of these practitioners specialise in the treatment of abdominal adhesions from a hands-on perspective and have years of experience treating patients.

Interview with Amanda Oswald

On myofascial release and visceral manipulation

What is fascia?

Fascia is the connective tissue that attaches, stabilises, encloses and separates all structures within the body, including muscles, bones, nerves, blood vessels and organs.

Most of the soft tissue in the body is a combination of muscle and fascia. Fascia wraps around all of the organs. It fills in the spaces and forms a three-dimensional network throughout the body. What is interesting is that fascia is also believed to be a communication system which can transmit messages much faster than the nervous system.

Amanda goes on to say, 'All viscera are wrapped in several layers of fascia'. The fascia can become restricted, resulting in dysfunction and hence the presentation of symptoms, either at the given location or at a distal point. These restrictions effect the body gradually and, in the case of the viscera form adhesions where organs may become stuck together. The body adapts over time, and it is this adaptation that can cause a situation where there is chronic pain.

Causes of fascial restrictions

Causes of fascial restrictions include surgery, accidents such as whiplash, falls, breaks to bones, repetitive movements or sedentary lifestyle. When fascial restrictions occur, the fascia loses its natural fluid nature and instead, becomes thicker and stickier, adhering together. The fascia thickens due to activation of fibroblasts within the fascia causing more collagen to be produced. As a result, the fluid within the tissues is squeezed out.

Stress is a major cause of fascial restrictions, Amanda says, but the cause of fascial restrictions are always multifactorial. Lifestyle factors, as well as injury, play a role.

Fascia holds onto emotions, and patients can release these emotions when undergoing treatment. This process is known as unwinding. With major unwinding, patients may respond with big physical movements, although for many people their releases are internalised. This is the mind and body, letting go of the stored emotion that was not previously processed.

Hands-on work

There are specific techniques that Amanda uses with hands-on therapy in order to provide relief from the restrictions that have formed. The fundamental aim of treatment is to release the restrictions. Amanda describes the fascial restrictions as feeling denser and more 'stuck down' and during treatment, there is a distinct change in the way the fascia feels as the restrictions are released.

Adhesions can also affect the viscera in the body, thus affecting their inherent natural rhythm. Indeed, fascial restrictions and adhesions can cause the viscera to become congested, and this congestion has widespread systemic effects. Myofascial release around the viscera will allow the organ in question to return to its normal rhythm. This is a concept found in visceral manipulation. The hands-on work can also help to release trapped nerves that play a role in pain present in these patients.

As fascia contains a lot of water, a damp heat environment can assist in melting restrictions. Movement is also highly recommended, and patients should keep active. They can regularly practice Qigong, Tai Chi, Yoga, Pilates etc. whatever the patient prefers.

Abdominal adhesions

Abdominal adhesions can form due to abdominal surgery. For example, if a patient has had part of their colon removed, the body will fill in that area with scar tissue, and this may continue to grow along natural lines of tension and eventually stick onto other internal structures. Amanda says, *'You can feel the scar tissue, you can feel the lumps'*. Patients can develop pain over the area of surgery, as the scar tissue can pull the fascia in a certain way. The issue here, is that patients can end up in a cycle of recurrent surgery as they attempt to resolve the pain caused by the adhesions. This is not ideal as more adhesions form with each operation.

With myofascial release, it is possible to break down the scar tissue and adhesions. You can feel a solid area of scar tissue decrease as it breaks down. It will go from one solid area, to several lumps, to grains of sand. This is felt through the treatments. The body reabsorbs the excess collagen, and as it does this, the scar tissue left in the affected area becomes more functional. There will always be a degree of scar tissue, but the main purpose of the treatment, is to return normal function to the body.

Preventing abdominal adhesions after surgery

Amanda can work on patients after surgery once the skin has healed. The myofascial release techniques that Amanda uses are gentle and not aggressive. The aim of the treatment is to mobilise the tissue in order to prevent major scar tissue forming, or shall we say the wrong type of scar tissue forming. Scar tissue that creates a problem is the type that creates patchwork repair, and in this case the collagen does not align with the fibres around it. Myofascial release can help with the healing so that the collagen that is laid down is more in line with the tissue around it.

Generally, six sessions are needed; once a week with exercises in between the sessions is generally enough time to see a lasting improvement, Amanda says.[224]

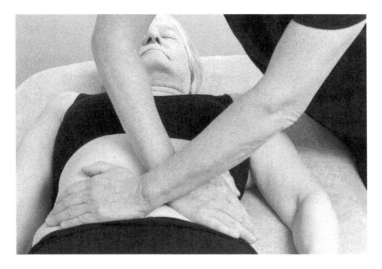

Figure 22. **Myofascial x-hand stretch for the abdomen:** this technique is useful for help-ing to release the layers of fascia that can become stuck in the abdomen leading to fascial restrictions that may affect digestion and general organ function. Photo and description, courtesy of Amanda Oswald—www.paincareclinic.co.uk.

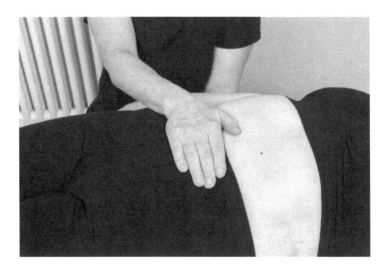

Figure 23. **Myofascial transverse plane release for the abdomen:** in this technique, the therapist 'sandwiches' the abdomen between their hands, allowing the energy flow between their hands to help release fascial restrictions—it is particularly effective to start the release of scar tissue and adhesions. Photo and description, courtesy of Amanda Oswald—www.paincareclinic.co.uk.

Interview with Marty Ryan

On myofascial release and visceral manipulation

Visceral manipulation and myofascial release are well used and poorly defined, Marty says.

'Visceral manipulation' is a brand name: it is a low force, light touch work, looking for and influencing a movement pattern that is endemic in our viscera. In visceral manipulation, extensive mobilisation does not occur. There is a specific meaning to the words visceral manipulation that Marty does not perform explicitly in his practice. He does manipulate the viscera, but he is not using visceral manipulation as his style of treatment.

Myofascial release is another tricky one, Marty explains, as there is facia everywhere. Everything is built around the facial network, and it is micro and macro.

With the style of manual therapy that Marty practices, he is absolutely changing the status of the visceral facia. Marty says, 'Every time we breathe we change something about how the large bowel is anchored, we move the upper abdominal organs into the lower abdominal organs. Everything moves all the time'. What Marty is doing is specifically meeting an organ he is choosing to work with and mobilising it and asking the nervous system to change holding patterns in order to create ease and therefore provide more movement. Marty does this in a way that involves more contact than visceral manipulation, but not in a rolling or deep high-pressure way either, because the viscera don't need that and respond poorly to it. With this type of work, it is important to use the right amount of pressure. The therapist needs the skill and technique to be able to feel exactly what they are doing and to be able to differentiate between the organs and structures that they are working on.

In Marty's experience from teaching these techniques, he finds that most therapists do not get this type of training. It is extremely important to develop the sensitivity and understanding of each layer of the facia and to know what you are feeling. Marty's favourite word to describe what he does is manual therapy. Its manual therapy that effects the viscera, facia and enteric nervous system. These three aspects of the body are so intimately related, especially when there is pain, tissue trauma, bloating and swelling.

Manual therapy also effects positive changes at the level of the autonomic nervous system. One of the signs, Marty says, that this is happening is borborygmus is escalating. This usually occurs in the first 5 minutes of treatment. Marty is able to feel the nervous tension in the tissues of the abdomen. He describes it as a sensation of hard armouring. The tissue feels hard at first, and then it softens and yields and allows more breath, blood flow and becomes more mobile. Armouring is a texture or signalling in the body that holds an emotion that is unfinished or unprocessed—this is how mind–body medicine describes it. Marty does not necessarily use it in this way, although he believes that one's emotional state can affect the abdomen and the viscera. In this context, Marty is using the word armouring, in holding, to define the texture.

Digestive disorders which respond well to manual therapy

GERD

Marty finds that acid reflux and hiatus hernia respond well to manual therapy. Acid reflux is a condition that is extremely prevalent worldwide. Marty believes that it is related to an autonomic nervous system dysfunction which compromises the function of the cardiac sphincter as well as the acid production.

From a manual therapy perspective, Marty is mechanically moving the stomach away from the diaphragm by hooking the lesser curvature of the stomach with his hands. The intension here is twofold. First, to manually make more space between the diaphragm and the cardiac sphincter. Second, to ease the tension in that region so that the three layers of smooth muscle relax and the autonomic nervous system changes its status from alarm to relaxed and is eased. As a result, better function occurs.

This does not mean that Marty is opening or closing the sphincter; it means that he is trying to normalise and balance the system. Marty can't actually touch the cardiac sphincter as it is under the rib cage, but he can hook, with his finger pads, the lesser curvature of the stomach in order to pull the stomach downwards. Marty sees tremendous results in patients suffering from reflux and hiatus hernia. He is amazed to see how quickly things change in as little as four to six sessions. Four to six sessions are enough for the patient to improve to such a degree that they are thinking of stopping their PPIs or taking a break from them.

Marty feels there are great tie-ins with internal medicine practitioners like herbalists and other natural medicine practitioners, as the two therapies complement each other very well.

Small intestinal bacterial overgrowth (SIBO) and constipation

Marty sees a lot of patients in his clinic who have been diagnosed with SIBO and constipation. In these cases, Marty's treatment plan is to change the status of the ileocecal (IC) valve. This increases the kinetic ability of the small intestine to move its contents through, thus improving peristalsis and preventing stagnation. This prevents the contents of the bowel sitting around and putrefying and releasing gases. Often times it is the IC valve that is holding things back and not allowing movement in a timely manner.

Marty says that SIBO and constipation are examples of conditions where it is important to work alongside natural medicine practitioners.

Abdominal adhesions

Abdominal adhesions do not always equal bowel obstruction, but in many cases, they do. Marty has worked with several patients who were diagnosed with bowel obstructions caused by abdominal adhesions with great results. The patients were able to move to a place where they were not having episodes of pain anymore.

What happens to the adhesions during treatment?

It really depends on the adhesions in question as to what is actually happening with treatment Marty says. Some adhesions are more superficial and very weak and easy to work on. Other adhesions are so adhered and stuck and thickened; some are even vascularised. In these cases, it would not be advisable to rip them as this could cause more tissue trauma. Some of the adhesions that are not well-formed and weaker in nature are delaminated by the treatment. The lysis of adhesions performed by surgical intervention even by keyhole surgery creates more tissue trauma as verified by many surgeons.

Some of the work Marty does, is to put the sticky, gluey adhesive tissue into tension, which then changes the nervous systems relationship to the affected area. For example, if two loops of the small intestine are stuck together, Marty will place his fingers into that space and attempt to move them apart. He will then move his fingers away, and the tissues will move back together. Marty will perform this action about eight to ten times in a session. Marty is certain that by performing this technique, he is speaking to the enteric nervous system. Marty also believes that by creating tension and release he is improving the mobility of the sticky, gluey adhesive material so that the bowel is less anchored and hardened and more mobile. As a result, the adhesion is stretched out, and there is more give.

The fact that these adhesions are present changes the function of the bowel. It is not complete dysfunction, but the dysfunction is significant enough to have consequences on the functioning of the digestive system. Sometimes obstruction occurs, and this is an issue. However, it is not only the adhesion's which cause problems, but the damage to the nerves and tissues caused by the surgery. All of this causes a change in the nervous systems acknowledgement of proprioception. As well as the trauma caused by the surgery, there is also the fact that the internal organs have been exposed to the atmosphere. This effects the tissue of the body.

How soon after surgery should treatment begin?

Marty recommends that patients start with manual lymph drainage at about 1 week after surgery. This type of treatment is much lighter and will help to improve the lymph drainage. Marty will then see the patient 4 weeks after surgery.

Marty has found that there are particular areas where adhesions form depending on the type of surgery performed. It is common for adhesions to form on the loops of the small bowels with abdominal surgery. When cholecystectomy is performed the duodenum will stick under the slot of the liver and the portal triad will stick to the duodenum. Marty can provide substantial relief in the upper right quadrant post-cholecystectomy. Marty has also seen many patients that have had total colectomies and there are adhesions everywhere in these patients.

Marty teaches these skills to physiotherapists in Europe who have not had training in this type of manual therapy. In this way, they are able to help patients suffering from adhesion-related problems. Marty says that teaching physiotherapists is probably the best integration point as they are well accepted in the mainstream medical model.[225]

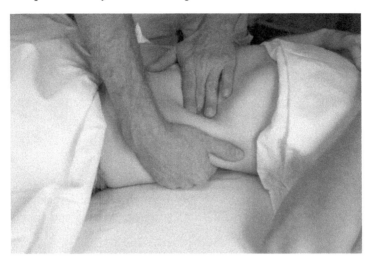

Figure 24. Here Marty is working with the descending colon. Lofting the bowel from the posterior side while compressing from the anterior side. Photo and caption courtesy of Marty Ryan—www.loveyourguts.net

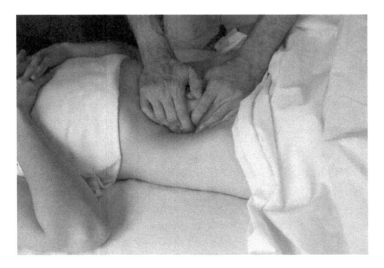

Figure 25. Here Marty is making his way through the loops of the small bowel to eventually meet the DJ flexure—where the duodenum meets the jejunum. Photo and caption courtesy of Marty Ryan—www.loveyourguts.net

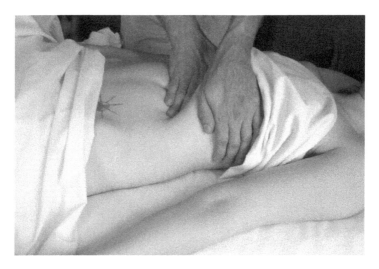

Figure 26. Here Marty is working with the greater curve of the stomach as well as mobilising the left rib margin and respiratory diaphragm. Photo and caption courtesy of Marty Ryan—www.loveyourguts.net

Interview with Isabel Spradlin

Why is activity in the form of exercise and stretching is so important when dealing with abdominal adhesions?

Isabel states, 'Whole-body activity is absolutely necessary to making progress with adhesion-related problems, but it is so individual'.

Movement is essential: our bodies are simply biologically made to respond to activity, Isabel says. There are all sorts of metabolic and central nervous system processes that are activated when we start moving that are essential to health.

When it comes to the abdominal contents, the abdominal organs and the abdominal muscles, they respond in much the same way, responding very well to movement. All of the organs within our abdomen are not free-floating; they are all tethered by their own ligaments and tendons. When tissues get stuck together, they have a hard time moving and sliding over each other as they should, and problems can start to develop. The hands-on work is a great way to start to release these restrictions and to help to restore normal function. The movement, the exercises and stretches, help in conjunction with the hands-on work to ensure these tissues that were previously adhered together stay released or assist in promoting further release. An integrated system of treatment is the best approach when dealing with abdominal adhesions. This is Isabel's overall perspective, as to why movement is so important.

Which exercises are best?

The specific exercises that Isabel recommends are tied into specific hands-on releases. Isabel recommends performing the hands-on techniques first, followed by the specific exercises or stretches recommended. Most of these are yoga-based. The reason they are coupled together as part of the same programme is that they don't just work together, they need each other, Isabel sates. Though there are some generic exercises and stretches that Isabel has put together; when treating patients in the clinic, Isabel may alter and adapt the exercises to the patient's specific needs, as each patient is unique.

As part of the ongoing treatment protocol, in between treatment sessions the patient will perform the hands-on work themselves and then perform the required exercises and stretches to facilitate the release and maintain freedom of movement in the abdominal region. If the patients are not able to attend the clinic, they can still use the self-help protocol, and Isabel is able to support them via skype sessions. As the patient progresses with the treatment, the exercises change in relation to the patient's needs. This will help maintain the freedom of movement in the tissues or assist in opening up a specific area a little more. Whether working in person or online with patients, Isabel sees the exercise part of the treatment plan as vital in assisting the hands-on work.

Fear of moving

It is very common for patients that have adhesions to become fearful of movement. When patients are in pain and distress, they don't want to move, as they are not sure what will trigger a flare-up of acute pain or obstruction. However, once patients start to use the online programme and start to get relief. Isabel often hears them say 'I should have kept moving in those years when I was too afraid to move'.

Sometimes the things that help can make patients feel a little worse, to begin with, but it is important to gauge that over time. The practitioner is there to help the patient calibrate the movement, so that they have the least amount of discomfort and the maximum amount of benefit. Isabel feels that the support of the therapist is very important in assisting with this. The patient needs someone to help and encourage them to take small steps at a time. This can help to short circuit the fear mechanism that keeps them from doing anything. It takes time to build confidence through experience. Isabel recommends that patients keep logs of how they feel before and after movements and activities. Recovery hardly ever goes in a smooth upward line. The logs help patients track the trajectory of their progress. A patient may experience pain again and get lost in the fear, but when they refer to their logs, they can see that they have actually been better for longer. They can see that there has been a much greater time between episodes of pain, so they are actually improving. This helps patients understand that they are progressing and it assists them in staying committed to the movement and treatment.

Post-surgical bowel obstruction

Isabel says, 'the effect of anaesthesia on our entire system is overlooked'. This is something we also see in endobiogenic medicine, in the functional biology blood test. There are specific hormone and autonomic nervous system changes that occur during and after surgery, as an effect of the anaesthesia and the trauma caused by surgery. One of the pathways affected is the HPA axis, and we see a substantial rise in cortisol levels. Post-operatively, cortisol can stay high for 6 to 8 weeks or longer in some individuals. As discussed previously, when cortisol is high, it exhibits an immunosuppressive effect. This is just one of the many changes that occur. Isabel goes on to say that anaesthesia slows down everything, so just coming back online fully, metabolically speaking, takes a long time. Isabel theorises that the effect of anaesthesia plays a role in post-operative bowel obstructions for this reason. Another factor linked to adhesion formation, especially with laparoscopic surgery is the use of CO_2 to inflate the intra-abdominal cavity. The CO_2 can dry out the tissue in the intra-abdominal cavity, thus increasing the risk of adhesion formation.

In addition to this, the instruments themselves used in the surgical procedure sliding through the intra-abdominal cavity along the various tissues can cause trauma. Furthermore, the incisions made change the tension patterns throughout the abdominal musculature. The abdominal muscles are used to contracting in a certain way. Once those muscles are cut, those tension patterns have been fundamentally altered. It can take a long time for those muscles to relearn how to do their work in this new way. They need to adapt to a new function. As these muscles are relearning, it can cause shifts in how the abdominal contents sit in the belly, and this is yet another factor relating to the abdominal pain seen in these patients.

It takes time for the body to adapt to a new way of functioning and it can take a while for the central nervous system to process all of this information and set up new patterns that are not driving pain and causing the spasm, Isabel says. However, the central nervous system won't resolve an adhesion on its own, and that's where the hands-on therapy comes into play. The whole body has to relearn how to function. Out of all the patients that Isabel sees, the patients that come to her with bowel obstructions get the most relief as this treatment works well for these patients.

Some patients can seem to be functioning well, and then all of a sudden can develop an acute episode of adhesion-related pain and present with bowel obstruction. In these cases, there are a couple of factors to consider. First, there can be dietary irritation and this may be low-key irritation. In Isabel's opinion, there is usually some kind of dietary component in the trigger of acute obstruction. Hence, it is important to identify any potential food intolerances and remove them. Second, obstructions that come on suddenly have actually been building for quite some time and patients are not aware that they are having some low-key distress. Isabel trains her patients to look for this and address it immediately by implementing the hands-on therapy and stretches so that it does not progress into a severe episode of pain. This is generally the hardest part as when a patient notices a niggle or low-grade pain, they are busy working or doing other tasks, and they find it hard to step aside and address it.

However, this is very important as it can stop severe spasm and obstruction from developing.

Hands-on work and scar tissue

There are two types of scar tissue, Isabel says. The scar tissue that forms on the surface of the skin that serves a specific function, for example, when you are cut. With this type of scar tissue, you are working directly with scar tissue in a steady and respectful way, trying to soften them and trying to get them fully integrated into the surrounding tissue. Most patients are shocked at how well their scars can integrate.

The other type of scar tissue is the sticky adhesive tissue formed internally, that, for example, joins two loops of small intestine together. Here you are trying to work the tissues free from each other and to bring full blood flow back to the areas where blood flow has been impeded. The treatment also works on the lymphatic system, which assists in cleansing the area of dead cells. In this case, you are not really breaking anything apart; you are de-globing the area for want of a better word. This helps the different layers of tissue slide more freely over each other. We can talk about stretching apart adhesions, breaking apart adhesions or breaking down adhesions. All of this can be accurate, but it depends on the situation. There are extreme versions of adhesions in the belly that are thick and well-formed, strong webs of adhesion that act as connective tissue that is not in the right place. In these situations, we are getting more into the realm of what people talk about when they say stretching or softening the adhesions. In Isabel's experience, these very strong webs of adhesion are harder to break down.

In these situations, the main focus will be to work on softening and stretching the adhesions in the belly. Again, in a gentle and respectful way; not in an aggressive manner. On some occasions, Isabel has felt a snap when the adhesion releases and this is followed by a rush of warmth to the area where blood flow comes rushing back. When this occurs, it has not caused any pain or discomfort to the patient, and it is usually unexpected, as the main focus is working on softening and stretching that material, not breaking it apart. Working with that level of adhesion does take longer, and you need to approach it with a little bit of a different mindset, as it is not just about making the tissues slippery anymore. You have this whole extra tissue in the belly that you are trying to get to a functional level. Sometimes this webbing can be felt, but it depends on the person. Every person's body can reveal things in different ways and at different times. Once the different layers of tissue relax and open up more can be felt. When this happens, you can get quite rapid results. When the tissues relax, Isabel is then able to feel the different restrictions in the belly. If patients are very protective and guarded, in relation to their abdomens, then it is harder. You may have to work for several sessions, just on the muscular structure of the abdominal wall, in order to help their nervous system calm down enough to allow a deeper exploration. This exploration gives valuable information as to what kinds of restrictions are present with each patient.[226]

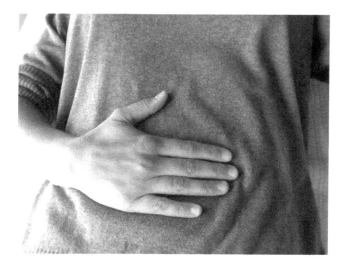

Figure 27. **Centre:** Begin and end by laying your hand(s) on your belly. Use your mind to help you breathe into your belly and to begin softening all of your tissues, including muscles, fascia, and organs. Use lots of imagination as you are getting used to the feel under your hands. Photo and caption courtesy of Isabel Spradlin—www.abdominaladhesiontreatment.com

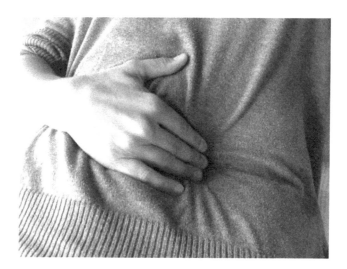

Figure 28. **Pull:** Gently begin to sink (do not push) your fingertips into your tissues. Keep your belly relaxed—all work is contained in the arm and hand. Go slow and don't try for depth right away. Imagine letting the deeper parts of your belly come to your hand. When you encounter uncomfortable spots, simply pause and see if the discomfort will decrease on its own. Photo and caption courtesy of Isabel Spradlin—www.abdominal-adhesiontreatment.com

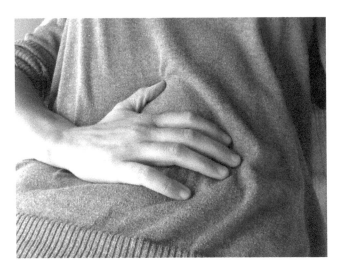

Figure 29. **Push:** Use the heel of your hand to gently sink (do not push) into the tissues of the other side of your belly. Keep your belly relaxed—all work is contained in the arm and hand. Imagine, and use, a gentle undulation from side to side in your belly, going from fingertips to heel of the hand, and back. This exercise is to increase the mobility of all of the tissues of the area, including the organs. Photo and caption courtesy of Isabel Spradlin—www.abdominaladhesiontreatment.com

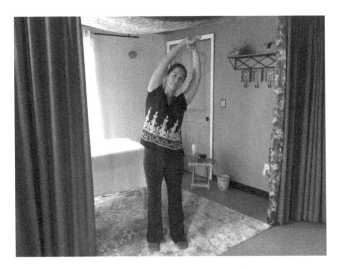

Figure 30. **Side stretch:** It is very common for the belly to become 'compressed' between the ribs and hips. Standing with your feet under hips, reach straight up to expand your belly. Stretch through the sides of your belly with a gentle bend to each side. Because the legs are often creating tension on the pelvis and belly, this is best-done standing to stretch them as well. You can also do it lying down or from a seated or kneeling position. Photo and caption courtesy of Isabel Spradlin—www.abdominaladhesiontreatment.com

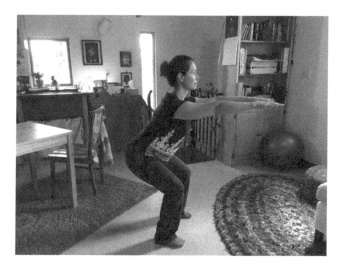

Figure 31. **Squat:** Strengthening your buttocks and legs is essential to releasing the tissues of the abdomen. If the abdomen is bearing all of the load of keeping you upright, it is sometimes difficult to get the tissues to fully release. Keep your knees behind your toes and squeeze your buttocks the entire time. Start slow and increase incrementally. Photo and caption courtesy of Isabel Spradlin—www.abdominaladhesiontreatment.com

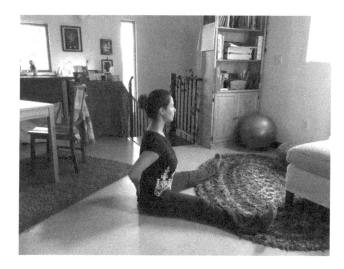

Figure 32. **Wide leg:** This is one of the best stretches I've found for both the pelvic floor and the health of the entire belly. Keep both sit bones grounded and your pelvis upright or neutral if you bend forward. Your legs do not need to start very far apart. Don't push the stretch too quickly. Stay comfortable. Sit on a bolster and use bolsters or rolled up blankets under your knees to modify and keep the stretch comfortable for yourself. Photo and caption courtesy of Isabel Spradlin—www.abdominaladhesiontreatment.com

CHAPTER TWENTY

Case studies

In this chapter, we will look closely at a variety of cases of digestive disorders, including Crohn's and colitis. The cases for each patient will be presented in detail, along with the findings of the endobiogenic clinical examination. For some of these cases, the functional biology results will be presented. This will depend on whether or not the patient had a functional biology test performed. The prescription, diet and lifestyle advice will also be presented with the rationale behind the advice given. We will be looking at the progress of each patient step by step as the treatment advances and the evolution of each prescription. This will help you understand the rationale behind the treatment.

With regards to the endobiogenic clinical examination:

A score of 1 to 5 is given in the form of a + symbol for each clinical finding where relevant. A score of 1 is the lowest, and a score of 5 is the highest.

Case 1

A 12-year-old male. Presenting with digestive problems for 2 months.
    Symptoms include: vomiting (sometimes for the whole week), bad breath, heartburn, loss of appetite. Only vomits in the morning then stops. Scared to eat. Stomach pain daily. Cramping sensation in the central abdominal region. Pain aggravated upon eating. Symptoms started 2 months ago with a vomiting bug. Is waiting for a referral to a gastroenterologist.

Investigations

- Ultrasound—all-clear
- Blood markers—nothing of note
- Negative for *H. pylori*

Medication: prescribed omeprazole by the GP

- No other medication given. GP said that he has anxiety.
- As he is constantly feeling ill, he is having to visit the school nurse. School have said that he is an attention seeker.
- Mother said he was always happy and positive as a child and only recently feeling down since ill.

Findings

- Hands cool ++
- Feet very cold ++++. When the feet are colder than the hands, it signifies that there is pelvic congestion
- Feet very damp ++++
- Large verruca on right foot. Two of them
- Splanchnic congestion ++++
- Blink response rapid +++
- Eyelids tremble a lot when closed ++++
- Adrenals congested ++++

Advice

- No sugar, gluten or dairy
- Lots of meat stock
- Stop omeprazole

Explaining the case

The chronic symptoms seen in this case were triggered by the vomiting bug. The terrain was in such a state that the pathogen (the aggressor) was able to induce a chronic state of imbalance resulting in the symptoms described. The organism was not able to adapt significantly to the aggressor and, i.e. return to its base level of functioning.

The aggressor brought into play, the syndrome of adaptation as any aggressor would. The autonomic nervous system was affected.

The bad breath is related to the alterations in the upper digestive flora and small bowel. Omeprazole can play a major role here as it triggers or worsens the dysbiosis as it suppresses and, in many cases, completely blocks stomach acid secretion. This causes, small intestinal bacterial overgrowth.

The question you may ask is, why was this patient not able to adapt successfully. Why did this patient end up with chronic symptoms and why were all the investigations from the hospital negative? Why do some patients clear the pathogen quickly and have no lasting symptoms but others, such as this patient, develop chronic symptoms?

The answer lies in the terrain. A patient who is affected in such a way and develops chronic symptoms has a specific pre-existing terrain that favours this. We have already spoken about pre-critical and critical terrain. This is why a thorough case history and specific physical examination is essential. The functional biology test is also an incredibly valuable tool in assessing the terrain. Bringing all of this information together allows one to devise an effective treatment plan.

Treatment plan

1. Reduce alphasympathetic activity, reduce parasympathetic activity, reduce splanchnic congestion, reduce TRH, support adrenals.
2. Restore gut microbiome and support the upper digestive system. Stop omeprazole as it is suppressing the stomach acid and impairing the digestive function, thus affecting the microbiome.
3. Prescribe an anti-inflammatory diet that will aid in the healing of the gut lining and remove the burden form digestive system. Use meat stock to nourish the lining of the digestive tract.

Treatment

Rx. 1

Gentiana lutea	10 ml
Centaurium erythraea	15 ml
Passiflora incarnata	20 ml
Carduus marianus	15 ml
Melissa officinalis	20 ml
Angelica archangelica	10 ml
Glycyrrhiza glabra 1:1	15 ml
Sig: 4 ml bid	105 ml

Rationale for prescription

Gentiana was chosen as it reduces parasympathetic activity. In addition to this its bitter qualities aid digestion. It is an interesting plant as, initially, when the compounds within *Gentiana* make contact with the tongue they act to increase parasympathetic activity, but once those compounds are in the stomach, they act to reduce parasympathetic activity. *Centaurium* as a bitter to assist digestion. *Passiflora* to reduce alphasympathetic activity. *Carduus* to support the liver, as a mild beta-mimetic and as a splanchnic decongestant. *Melissa* to relax the sphincter of Oddi and as a GABA-ergic plant. *Angelica* as an antispasmodic and digestive. *Glycyrrhiza* to support adrenals and reduce inflammatory activity as well as to help with the GERD. It is possible to reduce TRH indirectly by using alphasympatholytic plants, or you may choose to directly reduce TRH using something like *Fabiana imbricata*.

Rx.2

Green clay
Sig: 1/3 tsp bid soaked in a glass of water overnight. Stir and drink first thing in the morning 30 minutes before meals.
Green clay is used to help correct the dysbiosis, detoxify, reduce inflammation and assist in re-mineralisation.

Rx.3

Ulmus fulva (slippery elm) powder
Sig: 1 tsp tid in a little water after meals
Ulmus is used for its demulcent properties. This works well when dealing with GERD and helping patients come off of PPIs.

Rx.4

Lotion

Lavandula angustifolia EO	2 ml
Chamomilla recutita EO	1 ml
Calendula macerated oil	50 ml
Sig: apply to solar plexus tid	

Using an external application of essential oils can help tremendously. If the essential oils are used daily, they will absorb through the skin and have a systemic effect. *Lavandula* EO will reduce alpha significantly and will reduce para slightly, the *Chamomilla* EO acts to reduce alpha and para. It is also antispasmodic. In this case, if the parent is performing the massage with the lotion or simply applying it, there is the feeling of being cared for and nurtured which has a therapeutic effect and will elicit positive changes at the level of the endocrine and autonomic nervous systems.

Rx.5

Probiotics—prescript assist
Sig: ½ capsule od then 1 od am
To re-establish healthy gut flora.

Rx.6

Great lakes gelatine
Sig: 1 tablespoon in a glass of water bid
As a nutritive and to help heal the mucosa of the digestive tract.

Follow-up appointment 1 month later

Improved after 3 days of treatment. Had one flair up that lasted just 1 day. Mother feels it could be a reaction to the skin of the courgette.

- Pain has more or less gone. A little pain related to gas on occasion.
- Opens bowels daily and no constipation.
- Energy is much better.
- No vomiting apart from when had this reaction to the courgette.
- No more burning in oesophagus.
- Bad breath has gone.
- Good appetite. Eating well. Enjoying eating stews. Eating plain food, no spices.
- Only drinks water.
- Stopped omeprazole.
- Weight is good. Mother said he has gained a bit of weight.
- Has not had to see the school nurse at all.
- White patches present on nails. This can be linked to zinc deficiency.

His mother said he is completely different now. He is not worried about eating or going to school anymore. Before was in constant pain. He is sleeping well and feeling happy again.

- When his mother massages him with the lotion on his solar plexus and abdomen, he feels better straight away.
- He is still waiting for the referral to a gastroenterologist.

Treatment

Repeat all medication and also added in a multivitamin and mineral and zinc drops.

Follow-up appointment 2.5 months later

Developed viral gastroenteritis in January. This caused a relapse of gastrointestinal symptoms but settled quickly. Had some grumbling in the bowel at the time.

- Not having pain in abdomen now
- No flatulence

- Sleeping very well
- No reflux
- The verruca has gone
- Weight stable
- His mother says has an allergy to dust mites

Findings

- Hands not cold but very slightly clammy +

Treatment

Rx. 1

Ribes nigrum	15 ml
Glycyrrhiza glabra 1:1	10 ml
Centaurium erythraea	10 ml
Passiflora incarnata	20 ml
Juglans regia	15 ml
Melissa officinalis	20 ml
Angelica archangelica	20 ml
Sig: 4 ml bid	105 ml

Also, carry on with green clay, *Ulmus fulva* (slippery elm) powder, lotion, probiotics prescript assist, Great lakes gelatine, multi and zinc drops.

Rationale for prescription changes

Used *Juglans regia* as an intestinal drainer and antiseptic agent due to viral gastroenteritis. *Ribes* to further support adrenals and sustain beta activity.

I have followed this patient for many years. He is doing very well with no sign of any digestive issues. He has not required any herbal treatment in recent years.

Case 2

A 9-year-old female suffering from digestive problems. Symptoms include stomach ache, belching, acid reflux and headache. Has pain with lots of gas.

- Stomach ace is always present
- Symptoms started earlier in the year
- History of anaemia. Very pale

Last year lots of flatulence and belching. Flatulence not that smelly. Belching tastes of food and acid. Reflux had been getting worse over the last few months and now stable in its progression.

- When lying down reflux worse
- Took gluten out of the diet and seems to have helped
- Physical exercise seems to make it worse
- Nothing seems to help significantly
- *H. pylori*-negative and nothing to note on bloods
- No stool investigation performed

About 9–10 months ago, the problem got worse. At this time had problems with closest childhood friend. Was upset for a while.

GIT

- Pain in the upper epigastric region at night and sometimes in the day.
- Had an ultrasound in Germany all looked fine.
- Opens bowels once or twice daily. No blood. She says stools may look a bit reddish or yellowish. Diarrhoea but not often.

Past

- Colicky as a child. Colicky at a very young age and did see a chiropractor.
- Teething was very bad.
- Was not interested in eating solids for 3 years.
- No eczema or asthma.
- Tendency to mouth ulcers and verrucae.
- Mothers pregnancy fine. Birth was okay, born 2 weeks premature.
- Breastfed 2 months as mother had a job lined up. Fed formula milk after this and cow's milk.
- General immunity good.
- Antibiotics in the past but not too many.

Immunisations: all the usual ones. No immunisations recently.

Sleep

- Difficult to get to sleep. Can take 1.5 hours.
- When goes swimming falls asleep easier.
- When does fall asleep mother says is a very peaceful sleeper. When wakes is very tired. Takes a long time to get up in the morning. The last few months it has been harder to rise in the mornings.
- Does not always remember dreams.

Diet

Likes bread. Likes to eat a lot of fruit in the mornings. Grapes, apples, lots of potatoes. Eats lots of greens.

BF: gluten-free bread, honey and olive spread. Lots of melon.

Snack: banana, bread with honey and sometimes jam. Raisins, grapes, blueberries and melon.

Lunch: school food.

Afternoon snack: hummus, rice, peppers and cucumber, apples.

Dinner: potatoes, vegetables, green beans. Not much protein at the moment.

Findings

- Pancreas congested +++
- Liver not congested
- Cold feet and hands and damp ++++
- Eyelids tremble when closed +++
- Adrenals congested ++++
- Prolonged skin redness on rolling

Advice

Follow a grain-free diet.

Explaining the case

In this case, all the tests from the hospital are negative. There is no pathological problem here; rather, it is a functional problem related to a dysfunction of the autonomic nervous system. From the findings, we can see that there is substantial pancreatic congestion which will be implicated in the digestive disfunction. The feet and hands are cold and damp, and this is linked to the high alpha and para states. Remember that alpha is a constrictive system and plays an important role in the splanchnic congestion (in this case only over the pancreatic region) present. The patient is not able to digest the food she has eaten efficiently. The reflux is linked to the dysfunction of the cardiac sphincter caused by the imbalance in the autonomic nervous system. The sphincter is not closing as there is a loss of tonus due to the high para. There is a deficient peripheral beta activity which maintains the congestion as para and alpha are not being reset. There is a high central beta activity (TRH). The patient is very reactive and sensitive, and this can be seen by the worsening of her symptoms over the 9–10 month period when she had difficulties with her close friend.

The difficulty in getting to sleep is linked to the high central alpha and beta state. The swimming helps her to fall asleep, as the physical activity assists, to a degree, in the rebalancing of the autonomic nervous system by improving peripheral beta activity and reducing alpha activity.

Being tired in mornings and finding it hard to rise, implies a high para and a deficient peripheral beta activity. This is linked to an underactive adrenal gland. The patient does not always remember her dreams. This does not mean that there is a low TRH.

Poor dream recall can be due to the fact that a high para can block the dream recall. Hence, it is possible to have a high TRH and still not remember your dreams. The prolonged redness of the skin is linked to high histamine activity. Remember, histamine is the autacoid of alpha and histamine stimulates alpha and retards beta activity.

Treatment plan

1. Reduce alphasympathetic activity, reduce para, reduce central beta (TRH), decongest pancreas, support adrenals and reduce histamine.
2. Improve the microbiome of the gut.
3. Remove grains from the diet. This will help the microbiome and will also take the strain of the digestive system.

Treatment

Rx. 1

Ulmus fulva (Slippery elm) powder
Sig: ½ tsp tid in water on an empty stomach
Ulmus is used for its demulcent properties. This works well when dealing with GERD.

Rx.2

Suggested probiotic but said had kefir and would take that to replace probiotic.
To help rebalance the microbiome

Rx.3

Green clay
Sig: 1/3 tsp in water, od, am, on an empty stomach
Green clay is used as an anti-inflammatory for the GI system. It is also a fantastic detoxifier.

Rx.4

Lavandula angustifolia EO	0.5 ml
Gentiana lutea	5 ml
Chamomila recutita	15 ml
Glycyrrhiza glabra 1:1	10 ml
Filipendula ulmaria	10 ml
Elettaria cardamomum	10 ml
Angelica archangelica	5 ml
Sig: 20 gtt bid increase slowly to 50 gtt bid	50 ml

Rationale for prescription

Lavandula to reduce alpha and to relax the sphincter of Oddi. *Gentiana* as a bitter and to reduce para. *Chamomila* as an antispasmodic, anti-inflammatory and it also reduces alpha and para. *Glycyrrhiza* to support peripheral beta, anti-inflammatory and antacid. *Filipendula* as an antacid. *Elettaria* as a carminative. *Angelica* as a digestive antispasmodic and warming bitter.

Rx.5

Magnesium liquid
10 ml at night
As an antispasmodic and to support the nervous system as well as the many other benefits magnesium offers.

Follow-up 2.5 weeks later

- Has been feeling much better.
- Stomach pain has gone.
- No reflux when lies down now.
- Belching has reduced considerably, and flatulence has decreased. Much better now.
- Headaches still present. Has a headache every day. Feels like an ache over the head. Test for sinus pain positive. This is a basic test where you ask the patient to lean forward so that their forehead is parallel to the floor and hold it for a short while. If there is pain or if the pain worsens it is positive.
- Could not take clay as was gaging.
- Took a probiotic instead of kefir.

Sleep

- Magnesium has helped her settle at night but still too stimulated to relax and finds it hard to sleep.
- Tired in mornings.
- Overall though sleep is better.

Diet

- Cut out grains, no refined sugar. Less fruit and more veg.
- Increased her protein and fats. Avocados, nuts and having more chicken and eggs.

Treatment

Repeat all prescriptions apart from clay. The headaches should improve as the patient progresses with the diet and the longer she is on the herbal treatment. Once the autonomic nervous system rebalances and the pancreas is less congested, the sinus congestion will diminish.

Added in

Rx.6 to aid sleep and to reduce TRH
Leonorus cardiaca
Passiflora incarnata
Melissa officinalis
Equal parts
Sig: 20 gtt od noct

Follow-up 1 month later

- Belching has reduced to once a day.
- No abdominal pain.
- Opens bowels once or twice a day.
- Tendency to lose stools since started medicine. This is most likely due to the magnesium.
- Felt 50 gtt of Rx4 was a lot so advised 20–25 bid.
- Stools can be smelly. Is having flatulence when exercising (running) and can be smelly. Mother does not feel it is extreme.
- Headaches reduced to once a week now, not daily.
- Can have episodes of sneezing; possibly allergy related.
- Sinus pain test negative now.

Diet

- Has reintroduced some potato, a small amount only twice a week.
- Lost a little weight.
- Had pasta once and felt ill after.

Sleep: able to settle faster now.

Advice

Stay off gluten, sugar and dairy for at least 5 months. Can have a bit of potato if she wants.

Treatment

Repeat all medications.

Follow-up 3 months later

GIT

- No burping, no pain.
- Opens bowels once a day. No loose stools.
- Not much flatulence, only very little.
- Still careful with diet but not as strict as she was.
- Headaches much better, does not have severe pain now. No sinus pressure.

Finds it hard to let go of things, e.g. homework. Is a very sensitive person can't let go easily. Advised to look into CBT and mindfulness to help let go and deal with the anxiety that it causes.

Case 3

A 57-year-old male presenting with gastrointestinal problems. Contracted giardia 22–23 years ago. Since then, digestion has never been good.

Recently developed fatigue and needs to sleep in the afternoon. Fatigue started 6 months ago. Fatigue occurs in afternoons. Feels needs to sleep at 4 pm. Feels better after naps. No stress or problems. Feels does not get stressed.

History of high blood pressure, developed this 12 years ago. This occurred when started a new stressful job. Was on medication for 2 years then stopped medication as changed to a less stressful job. Does enjoy work now. Not stressed by it. Travels abroad often with work. Sometimes long flights. Does get jet-lagged but feels can sleep easily.

Now exercises three times a week to help reduce blood pressure. Exercise helps reduce blood pressure to 130/80 without exercise blood pressure is 160/100.

Medication

Aspirin as a precaution.

Family history: Lots of strokes in the family.

Sleep

- 10.45 to 11.30 pm in bed. Weekends 11.30 to 12.30 pm in bed.
- Falls asleep straight away.
- Sleeps through the night and up between 5–7 am.
- Does not always remember dreams.
- Can get up quite quickly in the mornings.

GIT

- Stools very loose or diarrhoea
- This occurs in waves, better then worse
- Says stools probably sink not sure
- Tenderness in left lower abdominal quadrant
- Stools not pale
- Occasional flatulence

Diet

Breakfast

- Porridge with milk, sometimes coconut milk or eggs, smoked salmon or just a banana. Has coffee with milk no sugar, two a day. Tea with milk.

Snack

- None. If does snack it is not often, has bounce balls. Cake not often.

Lunch

- Chicken salad or sushi

Dinner

- Fish and veg. Omelette and tuna, steak and veg.

No fizzy drinks. Has carbonated water daily. Drinks red wine.

Findings

- Blood pressure 122/80
- Cold feet ++
- Has athlete's foot and fungal infection on toenails
- Cool hands ++
- Damp hands +++
- Tenderness in the ileocecal region
- Splanchnic congestion ++++
- Adrenals congested ++++ can't lift skin

Advice

- Practice Tai Chi, autogenic training or other breathing techniques.

This is a very important part of the treatment. It can have an immensely beneficial effect in assisting with the rebalancing of the autonomic nervous system and even have beneficial effects on the endocrine system, if practised daily. For some reason, this is the part of the treatment advice that patients are least likely to follow.

Diet

- Cut out porridge, no dairy, no sugar, no grains, no fruit in the morning or after meals, no salads.
- Eat avocado if tolerated, steamed vegetables. No parsnip, no potato. Avoid kale for the beginning, stop bounce balls.
- Lunch and dinner. Eat any animal protein and vegetables only.
- Coconut oil 1 tsp three times daily as has high caprylic acid content so anti-fungal.
- If needed, can snack on backed apple and nuts if tolerated or avocado.
- Try to stop alcohol and coffee for 1 month to see how it feels.

Explaining the case

In this case, the giardia was the aggressor which initiated the disturbances present in the gastrointestinal system. In some cases, the aggressor may have been dealt with by the organism or with treatment, but the disturbances caused to the gastrointestinal system remain. This is because the aggressor was able to modify the terrain permanently, and the organism was not able to regain its normal level of functioning.

There most likely would have been specific imbalances in the terrain of the patient before contracting the giardia, which made him more susceptible to developing chronic gastrointestinal symptoms. This is why some patients may contract the same pathogen and not react in the same way, i.e. be able to re-establish normal digestive activity in a short period of time whereas other patients will develop chronic symptoms.

The aggressor affected the HPA axis, as is the nature of any aggressor and thus the adrenal cortex. Most likely, the fatigue is as a result of adrenal dysfunction, but the cause is not limited to this axis. There are many other causes of fatigue, and it is usually multifactorial; many pathways are implicated but some more than others or some as a result of primary imbalances. The microbiome is implicated and possibly the thyrotropic axis etc. However, we do not have a functional biology for this patient, so we are relying on case history and clinical examination findings.

The patient says that he does not get stressed. Many patients are under a lot of stress but are simply not aware of it. This is evident in the functional biology results of patients. Clinical examination findings: we can see that there is high alphasympathetic and parasympathetic activity. Para higher than alpha. Tenderness in the ileocecal region; remember that there are a lot of ACTH receptors in this region confirming the alphasympathetic activity. Splanchnic congestion is severe, which implicates the splanchnic organs; pancreas, spleen, gallbladder and liver. Remember, alpha is a constrictive system and plays a role in the congestion seen. Para is also implicated in the congestive phenomenon. Para bringing the secretions. The loose stools and diarrhoea are related to the high para, as para increased gut motility. Adrenal congestion is severe. There is peripheral beta insufficiency, so the autonomic nervous system cannot reset itself, thus maintaining the imbalance.

Treatment plan

1. Reduce alphasympathetic activity, reduce parasympathetic activity, decrease splanchnic congestion, especially decongest pancreas—remember its connection to parasympathetic activity, support adrenals.
2. Improve the microbiome of the gut and reduce gastrointestinal inflammation.
3. Modify diet, as suggested above. This will help rebalance the microbiome, assist in reducing gastrointestinal inflammation and take the strain off of the pancreas. Stopping alcohol will greatly assist in this. Stopping coffee will aid in adrenal recovery.

Treatment

Rx. 1

Probiotic; Optibacs *Saccharomyces boulardii*
Sig: 2 capsules bid increasing to 3 bid after 1 week
S. boulardii is a transient probiotic which will assist in cleansing the colon as well as reducing inflammation. It is a useful probiotic for cases of diarrhoea.

Rx. 2

Optibac probiotic high strength
Sig: 1 od am
To help correct the dysbiosis.

Rx. 3

Green clay
Sig: 1 teaspoon soaked overnight in a glass of water. Stir and drink first thing in the morning 30 minutes before breakfast.
Green clay is used as an anti-inflammatory for the GI system. It is also a fantastic detoxifier and anti-diarrhoeal.

Rx.4

Lavandula angustifolia EO	1 ml
Codonopsis pilosula	20 ml
Artemisia absinthium	5 ml
Juglans nigra	15 ml
Curcuma longa	20 ml
Chamomilla recutita	30 ml
Agrimonia eupatoria	15 ml
Sig: 5 ml tid or 7.5 ml bid	106 ml

Rationale for prescription

Lavandula as an alphasympatholytic and to relax the sphincter of Oddi; thus assisting in splanchnic drainage. *Codonopsis* as an adaptogen to assist in energy. *Artemisia* as an anti-fungal and anti-parasitic. *Juglans* as an anti-parasitic. *Curcuma* as an anti-inflammatory, *Chamomilla* to reduce para and alpha and inflammation. *Agrimonia* to support pancreas, anti-diarrhoeal and intestinal antiseptic. *Agrimonia* will reduce parasympathetic activity indirectly by supporting the pancreas.

Advised to use paragon for 1 month after 1 month of using prescription Rx.4. Paragon is a fantastic anti-parasitic formulation.

Follow-up appointment 2 months later

At the beginning of treatment, he was starting to feel a bit better; stools were improving, more formed. Also, fatigue improved a bit. Then had to travel for 1 month and got exhausted. Worked 7 to 1 am. Has to do this once a year.

Diet

- Was not good as was not in control of what he was eating. Had diarrhoea when away as diet was bad. Did not have any abdominal pain.
- Alcohol—did not make too many changes.
- I advised again to stop or reduce alcohol.
- Stopped coffee but lasted 2 weeks, on coffee again.

Sleep

- Bad at the moment.
- Still wakes early 4–5 am. Hard to sleep again. In France took herbal sleeping medication and melatonin. Will carry on with this now is in London.
- Managed to do a guided meditation app 20 minutes daily.

Advised to go back onto a strict diet and stop coffee.

Findings

- Hands still cool/cold but not too damp
- Tongue white-coated
- Athlete's foot

Treatment

Rx.1

Candiphase cream on feet for athlete's foot
Topical anti-fungal.

Rx.2

Paragon for 2 weeks
Anti-parasitic.

Rx.3

Optibac probiotics high strength
To help correct the dysbiosis.

Rx.4

Green clay
Sig: 1 tsp bid
Green clay is used as an anti-inflammatory for the GI system. It is also a fantastic detoxifier and anti-diarrhoeal.

Rx.5

Ribes nigrum   100 ml
Sig: 3 ml od am
To support adrenal function

Rx.6

Codonopsis pilosula	20 ml
Artemisia absinthium	5 ml
Hydrastis canadensis	20 ml
Curcuma longa	10 ml
Chamomilla recutita	30 ml

Agrimonia eupatoria	15 ml
Sig: 5 ml tid or 7.5 ml bid	106 ml

Rationale for prescription

Replaced the *Juglans* with *Hydrastis* as the paragon formula contains *Juglans*. Also, *Hydrastis* is a fantastic mucous membrane trophorestorative and effective anti-inflammatory.

Follow-up 6 weeks later

- Had a skin rash then went away and now has itchy skin with no rash
- Lasted 3 or 4 days is now feeling better
- Said GP will check him for primary biliary cirrhosis and will test thyroid function and check cancer markers
- All liver functions normal
- Fatigue is better in the last few weeks
- Athlete's foot has improved

Diet

Breakfast: Smoked salmon, eggs and avocado.
Snack: Hummus, rice crackers and tomato. Occasional dates.
Lunch: Smoked mackerel with taramasalata, tomato and ham.
Dinner: Fish or meet with veg. Salad occasionally.
Off gluten completely. Once every 2 weeks had cake.

GIT

- Stools still loose.
- Can open bowels up to four times daily.
- Stools can be light and not formed.
- Can be watery. Chronic loose stools since 22–23 years old.
- Never had colonoscopy.
- Stool sample 10 years ago. Had *blastocystis hominis*.
- Also, had malabsorption.

Treatment

- Rpt: *Candiphase* cream, green clay, *Ribes nigrum*
- Stop paragon now
- In 2 weeks add in high potency probiotics again
- Advised to follow the GAPS diet

Rx.5

Melissa officinalis	10 ml
Artemisia absinthium	5 ml
Hydrastis canadensis	20 ml
Plantago major	25 ml
Chamomilla recutita	30 ml
Agrimonia eupatoria	15 ml
Sig: 5 ml tid or 7.5 ml bid	106 ml

Rationale for prescription

Removed *Codonopsis* as fatigue had improved. Added *Melissa* as it is useful for relaxing the sphincter of Oddi, so will assist in splanchnic drainage and for its GABA-ergic properties. Added *Plantago* as an antihistamine due to skin itching. *Plantago* is also a good intestinal drainer.

Follow-up 2 months later

- All blood work from GP fine. No primary biliary cirrhosis.
- Still had itching on the skin so saw a dermatologist. Dermatologist thought it was seborrheic dermatitis. Prescribed creams but did not use them.

Diet

- Followed GAPS diet fully for 3 weeks.
- Initially constipated for 1 day. No blood and no mucus.
- When stopped, the clay bowel motions returned.
- After 3 weeks stopped diet as had to travel and stools started getting loose again.

Advice

- If cannot follow GAPS diet when travelling I advised to completely avoid sugar, gluten and dairy.
- Decrease alcohol as much as possible.
- Follow GAPS where possible.

Findings

- Still lots of pancreatic, liver and adrenal congestion.

Treatment

Repeat green clay, probiotic

Rx.3

Ribes nigrum	100 ml
Cinnamomum zeylanicum EO	3 ml
Chamomilla recutita EO	2 ml
Boswellia EO	2 ml

Sig: 3 ml od am. Increase the dose slowly.

Rationale for prescription

Ribes to support adrenals. *Cinnamomum* EO for its antiseptic effect, and in EO form it supports adrenal cortex. *Boswellia* EO as an anti-inflammatory.

Rx.4

Curcumin x 4000
Sig: 2 am and 1 pm
As an anti-inflammatory.

Rx.5

Digestive enzymes
Sig: 1 tid with food start taking them in 2 weeks' time
To support the pancreas. By supporting the pancreas, you can indirectly reduce the overactivity of the parasympathetic nervous system.

Follow-up 1 month later

GIT

- Stools not as loose. They are now becoming more formed.
- Mainly float but sometimes sink.
- Stools are about 30% better. Definite improvement.
- A little flatulence.

Skin

- Is having a patch test on the skin to check for allergens.
- Itchy skin has resolved and not returned.

Diet

- Trying to have broth when can.
- No sugar, no dairy.

- On a low-carb diet. No bread and no pasta, no potatoes.
- Typical meal would be meet and veg.
- Feels is disciplined with diet now.
- Problem eating is on aeroplanes.
- Feels energy is good when has broth and follows GAPS diet. Energy is at its best when follows GAPS diet. Usually gets a 3 or 4 pm dip in energy but not when he has bone broth and meat stock.

Treatment

Repeat the same prescriptions as before.

Follow-up 2 months later

- Shortly after the last consultation, bowels improved more. Now has normal bowel movements for the first time in years. Had a bit of a flare-up when working. However, feels 6 out of 10 now. 10 is best.
- Wife says stools are not smelling as much now.
- Athlete's foot flared up recently.
- Had yellow fever jab and antimalarial tablets for 2 weeks as went to Africa over Christmas.
- Itching on the body has not returned.

Diet

- No alcohol since New Year, no sugar, no wheat and no dairy. Only little fruit.
- Having lots of avocado and broth when can.

Findings

- Tongue white-coated
- Pancreatic congestion better +++
- Liver congestion better than pancreas but still some congestion ++
- Tenderness in the ileocecal region better but not gone
- Adrenals much better can lift skin when rolling now

Treatment

Repeat Green clay, *Curcumin* x 4000, Rx.3, digestive enzymes and probiotics.

Added in

Zinc citrate 30 mg 1 with dinner and Renew Life Intestinew powder to help with healing of gut mucosa. Also, citricidal (grapefruit seed extract) as an anti-fungal.

Case 4

A 24-year-old female, presenting with digestive problems. Four years ago, had a lot of stress and developed IBS. Current symptoms include nausea and vomiting, acid reflux, abdominal cramping, loose stools and strong sensitivity to most foods. Feels anxiety is a problem. Stomach sore upon waking. Had severe episodes of vomiting that led to hospitalisation. Exploratory surgery performed with no problems discovered. The routine removal of the appendix at the same time as the exploratory surgery. Developed septicaemia post-surgery.

Currently, a university student and this has been stressful; soon to start a new job and looking forward to this. Previously when stressed has taken valerian and found this to be helpful. Smokes cigarettes and cannabis.

Endoscopy and colonoscopy results were normal. However, the patient informed me that the consultant mentioned that there could be a possibility of delayed gastric emptying. At this time prescribed antiemetic, antispasmodic and PPI medication.

Historical eczema has improved in the previous 6 months. No recurrent infections throughout life. Exercises twice a week with a personal trainer.

Medication

- Amitriptyline, 1 od
- Buscopan, prn
- Pantoprazole, prn

Supplements

- Megaspore biotic
- Slippery Elm capsules, 2 capsules od

Sleep

- 9 pm–2 am in bed.
- Takes time to fall asleep. Light sleeper.
- Does not remember dreams.
- Wakes at 8–11 am; feels groggy in mornings. Hard to rise.
- Did smoke cannabis in the past. Stopped approx. 6 months ago and since then energy in the day time is better.

GIT

- Opens bowel 2–3 times daily
- No constipation

- Loose stools
- Smelly flatulence

Periods

- Painful periods
- Occasional clots, not often
- January 2017: removal of ovarian cyst, right side
- September 2017: removal of a cyst, left side

Diet

- Eats little due to digestive symptoms present. Has tried to modify diet, no wheat, sugar or dairy.

Findings

- Hands cold ++
- Feet colder than hands +++
- Damp hands and feet +++
- Adrenals congested ++++
- Some generalised abdominal tenderness
- Eyelids do not tremble when closed. Patient may be squeezing eyelids too tight so hard to see
- Glabellar tap; little blink response; may be controlling the response
- Tongue white ++++

Functional biology results provided in table form

These are not all of the functional biology indexes. I have selected the most relevant ones related to this case. There are over 150 indexes. As discussed in Chapter 15, there is a Structure (S) value and a Function (F) value. The normal range for each index is listed in the last column.

Table 25. Shows the initial results before the start of treatment

Index	Initial results	Normal range
Beta MSH/alpha MSH	S 0.52 F 0.52	6–8
Cortisol	S 14 F 13.47	3–7

(Continued)

Table 25.(Continued)

Index	Initial results	Normal range
Adrenal gland activity	S 9.14 F 8.46	2.7–3.3
Permissivity	S 0.65 F 0.63	0.45–0.8
Peripheral serotonin	S 42.85 F 41.24	1.5–7.5
Cata-ana ratio	S 5.50 F 5.29	1.8–3
Inflammation	S 95.32 F 99.65	0.3–2.5
Genital estrogens	S 0.02 F 0.02	0.12–0.16
Genital androgens	S 0.02 F 0.02	0.12–0.17
Thyroid metabolic	S 0.46 F 0.46	3.5–5.5
Splanchnic congestion	S 1179 F 920.6	0.011–0.163
Insulin	S 117.4 F 113	1.5–5

Explaining the case

Case history and clinical examination

From the clinical examination, we can see that there is evidence of a high alphasympathetic and a high parasympathetic activity. The fact that the feet are colder than the hands signifies pelvic congestion. The adrenal glands are implicated in the imbalance of the organism as seen by the adrenal congestion present. The functional biology results which are available for this case will give details of exactly what is occurring with the adrenal glands. Remember that the act of vomiting is linked to a discharge of betasympathetic activity in an abrupt manner. In such patients, it is common for there to be a generally low peripheral beta activity, but as it builds over time this can discharge abruptly, causing vomiting. The acid reflux, nausea, loose stools and abdominal cramping are all linked to autonomic nervous system dysfunction as discussed in detail previously in the book. There is evidence of dysbiosis, and colon congestion as the patient has a white tongue. The generalised abdominal tenderness is linked to irritation/inflammation of the bowel. Cysts are linked to high FSH activity. Clots are linked to relative low progesterone to oestrogen ratio.

What is important, in this case, is to consider abdominal adhesions. This patient has had exploratory surgery, removal of her appendix and two operations to remove ovarian cysts. It is highly likely that abdominal adhesions will be present.

Functional biology

Coticotropic axis: The functional biology results, as seen in Table 25, confirm that there are indeed imbalances in the corticotropic axis. There is a significantly high cortisol activity, double what it should be, with overactivity in the adrenal gland. The permissivity index in this case is normal, but as the cortisol index is elevated, it means there is relatively greater maladaptive to permissive cortisol. Beta MSH/alpha MSH ratio is low showing there is relatively high alphasympathetic to betasympathetic activity. The peripheral serotonin index is substantially elevated as a result of stress on the organism. This index represents peripheral serotonin, and when elevated signifies a low brain (central) serotonin. This patient is more catabolic than anabolic as seen by the cata-ana ratio, which is in part, as a consequence of the elevated catabolic hormone cortisol. There is huge splanchnic congestion related to the autonomic nervous system dysregulation and thus, bringing all of the problems associated with it. Please refer to Chapter 5 on drainage.

Somatotropic axis: In relation to the somatotropic axis, we can see that insulin is extremely high and is a major factor in the inflammatory activity present in this patient. When the inflammation index is elevated, we must always look for the cause of the inflammation. In this case the insulin.

Gonadotropic axis: The gonadotropic axis reveals that there is a relative hypo functioning of the gonads with low genital oestrogen and androgen indices.

Thyrotropic axis: The thyrotropic axis indicates a low thyroid activity. This is linked to the blocking effect of cortisol. Remember, initially cortisol in its permissive role increases thyroid activity, but chronically elevated maladaptive cortisol suppresses thyroid activity. In addition to this, imbalances in the gonadotropic axis also affect thyroid activity.

In this patient, there isn't a huge difference between structure and function. In some patients, there can be extreme differences. With some, improving drastically when functioning and others improving when in structure.

Treatment plan

1. Reduce alphasympathetic activity, reduce parasympathetic activity. Support adrenals and reduce maladaptive cortisol levels.
2. Normalise cata/ana ratio by reducing cortisol.
3. Drain pancreas and support its activity.
4. Sustain peripheral thyroid activity.
5. Symptomatically reduce inflammation.
6. Reduce insulin.

7. Support gonads.
8. I did not choose to address the low central serotonin in the first month of treatment. I usually use 5-HTP to increase central serotonin, and some patients feel a bit nauseous with it. Given the patient's history of nausea, I did not prescribe it initially.
9. Though I have not specifically mentioned the need to reduce pelvic congestion in this case; by reducing FSH and rebalancing the autonomic nervous system, the pelvic congestion will improve. High FSH activity is a factor that contributes to an increase in pelvic congestion.

Advice

- Request vitamin D and liver function tests from GP.
- To follow the sugar-free, gluten-free, dairy-free and caffeine-free diet that I use in my clinic, as specified on page XX.

Treatment

Rx. 1

Megaspore biotic probiotic
Sig: 2 od for 3 weeks, then 1 od thereafter
To correct intestinal dysbiosis.

Rx. 2

Vitamin D
Sig: 2000 IU daily
To assist in reducing inflammation and for the many other benefits of vitamin D. Maintenance dose used until blood results are obtained. Also, some patients have a genetic polymorphism and can't tolerate large doses of vitamin D.

Rx. 3

Slippery Elm
Sig: 1 tsp tid
As a gastrointestinal anti-inflammatory.

Rx. 4

Planet paleo pure collagen
Sig: 1 scoop bid
To assist in the healing of the mucosa of the gut.

Rx.5

Agrimonia eupatoria	20 ml
Vitex agnus-castus	10 ml
Angelica archangelica	20 ml
Avena sativa	20 ml
Malva sylvestris	15 ml
Ribes nigrum	20 ml

Sig: 5–7.5 ml bid

Rationale for prescription

Agrimonia was used as an anti-diarrhoeal, anti-inflammatory and pancreatic drainer. By supporting pancreatic activity *Agrimonia* helps to indirectly reduce parasympathetic activity. *Vitex* to reduce FSH activity. *Angelica* as a digestive antispasmodic and for its mild oestrogenic effect. It helps to sustain gonadic activity. *Avena* to drain and support thyroid and for its mild oestrogenic activity. *Malva* to reduce insulin activity. *Ribes* to support adrenals.

Rx.6

Medi Herb Valerian Complex
Sig: 1 bid
To reduce alphasympathetic activity.

Rx.7

Pure encapsulations magnesium glycinate
Sig: 1 bid and increase to 2 bid in a week
To support the nervous system. Magnesium is also very useful for period pain and in the management of spasm. Glycine can also assist in the healing of the mucosa. I advised to increase slowly as too much magnesium can cause loose stools.

Follow-up appointment 1 month later

Reports improved energy and improved mood. It is now easier to wake in the mornings, feels more alert. Stomach less sensitive and not as easily affected by foods. No acid reflux; no longer experiencing cramps or spasms in the gut. No instances of vomiting or nausea.

- Has ceased smoking cigarettes for 3–4 weeks as well as cannabis
- Eczema, brief flare-up
- Has stopped taking amitriptyline

Sleep

- Improvements in sleep; falls asleep easier and sleeps deeper.
- Some vivid nightmares whilst reducing cannabis use, but has since improved.

Diet

- Followed diet sheet, eating regular portions of food.
- Now eating breakfast; unable to previously due to acid reflux. Is having porridge with almond milk or egg whites with spinach and mushroom.

GIT

- Daily bowel movements. Passing stools that are more formed than previously. Occasionally loose, but a definite improvement.
- Brief episode of constipation whilst on holidays, after flying.
- Flatulence improved; occasionally, some flatulence at night and a little smelly.

Periods

- Reduced period pain; feels 'much better'.

Treatment

- Repeat all supplements
- Added in 5-HTP to increase central serotonin
- Sig: 1 bid

Follow-up appointment 2 months later

Now working full time and enjoying it. Good mood has maintained, and others have noticed this. Her mother said that she is now a completely different person. Feels she is more resilient to stress.

There has been no recurrence of abdominal pain or discomfort and describes symptoms overall as 'much better' and mostly gone. No return of acid reflux, nausea or vomiting.

- Eczema flare-up on stomach and elbows.
- Still using valerian complex, vitamin D, slippery elm and collagen. Not using probiotics so much as felt they gave her acne on the face.
- Still off cigarettes and cannabis.

Sleep

- Further improvements in sleep quality
- No vivid nightmares

GIT

- Daily bowel movements; passes stools up to three times daily
- Stools are formed now
- Reduction in flatulence

Periods

- Regular; no clots now
- First 2 days are painful; less pain on days 3–5
- Heavy flow for the first 2 days

Treatment

Repeat slippery elm, collagen, vitamin D, valerian complex.
Advised to try a different probiotic to see if still has the same reaction with regards to acne. Try prescript biotic and increase the dose slowly.

Rx.5

Thyme vulgaris ct. *linalool* EO	0.5 ml
Citrus aurantium ssp. *aurantium* (Petitgrain) EO	1 ml
Ribes nigrum	25 ml
Avena sativa	20 ml
Angelica archangelica	15 ml
Smilax ornata	15 ml
Malva sylvestris	15 ml
Vitex agnus-castus	10 ml
Sig: 7.5 ml bid	

Rationale for prescription

Carried on with *Angelica*, *Avena*, *Malva*, *Ribes* and *Vitex* for the reasons mentioned above. Added *Smilax* to assist with eczema. Added *Thymus* EO mainly for its ability to reduce parasympathetic activity. *Petitgrain* EO to reduce alphasympathetic activity.

Follow-up appointment 5 months later

Eczema

- Not as bad now; there has been an improvement

Sleep

- No nightmares
- Not able to sleep well the past week, possibly due to work stress

GIT

- Overall good; apart from last week—possible virus; vomited one night.
- No spasms/cramps.
- Opens bowels daily: mainly twice daily. Once in the morning and once at night. On occasion opens bowels three times a day.
- Formed stools.
- Flatulence improved.

Periods

- Regular
- First 2 days remain painful

Findings

- Hands and feet a little damp ++ and cool +
- Feet not colder than hands now
- Adrenals congested +++
- No abdominal tenderness
- Eyelids tremble +++
- Glabellar tap; blink response rapid +++
- Tongue white ++

Repeat functional biology blood test 8 months after the start of treatment.

Table 26. Shows the results after 8 months of treatment

Index	Initial results	Results after 8 months of treatment	Normal range
Beta MSH/alpha MSH	S 0.52	S 3.30	6–8
	F 0.52	F 3.30	

(Continued)

Table 26. (Continued)

Index	Initial results	Results after 8 months of treatment	Normal range
Cortisol	S 14 F 13.47	S 6.75 F 6.24	3–7
Adrenal gland activity	S 9.14 F 8.46	S 6.88 F 5.88	2.7–3.3
Permissivity	S 0.65 F 0.63	S 1.02 F 0.94	0.45–0.8
Peripheral serotonin	S 42.85 F 41.24	S 10.42 F 9.63	1.5–7.5
Cata-ana ratio	S 5.50 F 5.29	S 3.86 F 3.57	1.8–3
Inflammation	S 95.32 F 99.65	S 3.49 F 3.84	0.3–2.5
Genital estrogens	S 0.02 F 0.02	S 0.09 F 0.10	0.12–0.16
Genital androgens	S 0.02 F 0.02	S 0.07 F 0.08	0.12–0.17
Thyroid metabolic	S 0.46 F 0.46	S 3.21 F 3.21	3.5–5.5
Splanchnic congestion	S 1179 F 920.6	S 6.03 F 3.57	0.011–0.163
Insulin	S 117.4 F 113	S 8.28 F 7.65	1.5–5

Follow-up functional biology results show substantial improvements in many markers.

Progress of the case

Clinical examination

From the clinical examination, we can see that there has been a reduction in the adrenal congestion, less dampness of the hands and feet so less parasympathetic activity. The hands are not as cold, so less alphasympathetic activity. There is no abdominal tenderness present now. Eyelids do tremble when closed now. This was hard to see when initially examining the patient and something to note. This could have been because the patient was squeezing their eyelids closed and not gently closing their eyes. This will affect the results of the examination. When examining a patient, it is easy to miss a sign and, i.e. it is very important to cross-reference with the information from the case history, as well as information from the functional biology. When the eyelids tremble when closed it signifies high TRH activity and this makes sense due to the initial complaint of anxiety. The tongue is still white, which implies colon congestion and fungal issues.

Functional biology

Corticotropic axis: The functional biology results, as seen in Table 26, confirm that there has been substantial improvement. The cortisol index is now completely normal. Adrenal gland and peripheral serotonin activity have vastly improved. The fact that the peripheral serotonin index has reduced means that central serotonin levels have increased. The Beta MSH/alpha MSH ratio has increased, meaning that there is now more betasympathetic to alphasympathetic activity. There is now more permissive activity, as demonstrated by the increase in the permissivity index. These results are in keeping with what the patient reports in the follow-up appointments. She feels calmer, her mood has improved, and she feels more resilient to stress. The splanchnic congestion has improved, so there is better drainage of the splanchnic organs and, i.e. better digestion. Lastly, the cata/ana ratio has improved as cortisol has reduced, so there is less catabolism.

Somatotropic axis: In relation to the somatotropic axis, insulin has dramatically reduced and is now approaching normal levels. Subsequently, there has been a reduction in inflammatory activity from 95.32 to 3.49 in structure.

Gonadotropic axis: An improvement in the genital oestrogen and androgen indices.

Thyrotropic axis: There has been a vast improvement in the thyroid metabolic index from 0.46 to 3.21 in both structure and function. These improvements are related to the reduction in the cortisol index.

This patient is still under my care and is doing very well.

Case 5

A 64-year-old male presenting with digestive problems. Diagnosed by his doctor as having gastro-oesophageal reflux disease (GORD). Symptoms include bloating after eating and epigastric discomfort. Developed GORD at age 21 and was diagnosed with an ulcer. Patient not sure if it was gastric or duodenal. At the time he also had a colonoscopy. Colon all-clear.

2002: ongoing personal life stress for 5 months that coincide with the return of his digestive problems.

Endoscopy resulted in the prescription of omeprazole. Took for 10 years, then ceased due to negative side effects (low libido, feeling 'strange' in the head/drowsy, pins and needles sensation all over the body). Upon cessation of omeprazole, negative side effects improved a little. Then developed a cough that improved with time. When not on omeprazole GORD returns.

Current symptoms include a feeling of pins and needles all over the body but not as severe as in the past, muscular pain in both legs, epigastric discomfort, bloating, abdominal cramp down both sides of the abdomen that can last 1–2 hours combined with back pain. Three weeks ago, experienced severe gut pain whilst taking a course of antibiotics.

Past

- Contracted gonorrhoea approx. 30 years ago that has resulted in the loss of physical sensation that impacts on sex. History of recurrent urine infections—treated with antibiotics.
- The patient states that antibiotics were useful in relieving the back pain associated with the UTIs.
- Two years ago, ongoing tooth infection—treated with antibiotics. Caused gut disturbance and pain. Felt better once the antibiotic course was completed.
- Used to experience significant pain when opening bowels. Can experiences pain and coughing following physical touch (e.g. massage).

Medications

Omeprazole
Sig: prn

Family history

N/A

GIT

- Regular flatulence which can be smelly
- Pain when passing stools
- No burning sensation in the stomach; GORD is the main problem

Diet

- High sugar diet; pastries and 5–6 chocolate bars daily
- Fizzy drinks, up to five colas daily
- Lots of bread

Findings

- Feet cold ++
- Damp feet and odorous +++
- Hands cold ++
- Abdominal pain and tenderness in ileocecal region ++++

- Liver and pancreatic (splanchnic) congestion ++++
- Adrenals congested +++
- Eyelids tremble when closed ++++
- Glabellar tap; blink response rapid +++
- Tongue white-coated

Advice

- To follow the sugar-free, gluten-free, dairy-free and caffeine-free diet that I use in my clinic, as specified on page XX.
- Patient will gradually reduce the amount of omeprazole.

Presenting the case

This patient has a long-standing history of upper digestive issues. There are most likely multiple imbalances present and testing for these would be advisable. However, the patient was not in a position to be able to have testing.

The alphasympathetic system is heavily implicated and part of the mechanism of ulcer formation that formed many years ago. The alphasympathetic system causes vasoconstriction, and when this occurs there is a lack of circulation and oxygenation to the tissue. With GORD there is a dysfunction of the lower oesophageal sphincter (LES) which is related to dysfunction of the autonomic nervous system. The LES loses its tonus, and hence reflux occurs. It is important to consider reducing parasympathetic activity here, as when it is elevated it relaxes the LES and reflux can occur. It would be advisable for the patient to have an endoscopy in order to determine if the ulcer is still present and to rule out a hiatus hernia.

There is also strong evidence linking low stomach acid to reflux. Many patients when tested are actually found to have low stomach acid as opposed to high. When this occurs the LES dilates causing reflux. I have had success using HCL supplementation in patients with acid reflux. Before using HCL, it is important to determine whether or not, an ulcer or gastritis is present as the HCL could cause irritation. Even if using HCL to treat low stomach acid, it is still important to try to identify the causes of the low acid.

This patient consumes a large quantity of refined sugar and has been doing this for a very long time. There are most likely issues lower down in the digestive system that could be disrupting the LES sphincter. We must also consider the fact that he has been on long-term PPI medication which is known to cause SIBO. Due to long term use of PPIs there is most likely malabsorption, and so mineral and vitamin deficiencies will be present which are often part of the cause of many strange symptoms.

The pain and coughing following physical touch demonstrate the hypersensitive nature of the patient. Regular flatulence means we need to consider supporting the pancreas and deal with any dysbiosis and possible fermentation that is occurring in the bowel.

The clinical examination shows that there is a high parasympathetic activity (damp feet) and alphasympathetic (cold feet, cold hands and rapid blink response). The congestion over the adrenals demonstrates the involvement of the adrenal glands in the autonomic dysfunction. There is tenderness and most likely inflammation of the bowel, especially where the ileocecal region is. Remember, this region is rich in ACTH receptors. Severe splanchnic congestion, will impair drainage of the splanchnic organs, thus effecting digestive activity.

There is high TRH activity. TRH affects the pancreas, stimulating insulin secretion. The constant sugar cravings can be triggered by high insulin and the need to fuel the constant mental activity (TRH). This would need to be confirmed with the functional biology results, but it is not possible at this time. The white-coated tongue signifies colon congestion and fungal issues.

Treatment plan

- Reduce inflammation, soothe and heal the gastrointestinal tract.
- Reduce para and alpha; alpha more so.
- Drain and support pancreas.
- Support upper digestive activity.
- Improve microbiome.
- With the history of ulceration, I wanted to start gently with treatment to see how it is tolerated.

Treatment

Rx. 1

Green clay
Sig: ½ tsp bid
To soothe and heal the gastrointestinal tract, starting with the oesophagus. Green clay is highly beneficial for any kind of ulceration of the gastrointestinal system.

Rx. 2

Slippery elm
Sig: 1 tsp tid pc
As an anti-inflammatory and demulcent to assist with the GORD.

Rx. 3

Gentiana lutea	10 ml
Centaurium erythraea	20 ml
Passiflora incarnata	20 ml
Sig: 2–3ml bid	

Rationale for prescription

Gentiana in order to reduce parasympathetic activity and is a valuable bitter, supporting upper digestive activity. *Centaurium* as a bitter to support upper digestive activity. *Passiflora* as an alphasympatholytic plant.

Rx.4

Optibac Extra Strength probiotics
Sig: 1 od am
To assist in correcting the microbiome of the gut. Recommended these as they do not contain FOS. In many patients the FOS can irritate their intestines

Follow-up appointment 2 months later

- Improvement in digestion.
- Less abdominal pain and spasm.
- Improvement in bloating. Less severe and less frequent.
- Less back pain.
- Reduced muscular pain in legs, compared to before.
- There has been significant pain in the epigastric region, approx. every 3 days; feels dizzy with the onset of pain. Pain seems to worsen a day after sexual activity as does oesophageal pain; takes omeprazole for this 2–3 times weekly. Only in presence of pain.
- Upon waking, the patient sometimes experiences numbness in one hand
- Over the past few days experiencing sharp pain in the left side of the groin and pain in the forearm when gripping something.

Diet

Patient reports he has followed diet advice. Reduced sugar and fizzy drink intake. Reducing dairy milk.

- Breakfast: 1–2 biscuits, cereal bar, black tea with honey
- One coffee daily, with one sugar
- Snack: banana or sardines
- Lunch: avocado, potato, salad, spinach, tuna and a few sips of fizzy drink
- Snack: cereal bar
- Dinner: grilled steak, mashed potato no butter, mixed veg
- Some bloating; occurs following milk consumption.

Advice

Advised patient to eliminate coffee, sugar, dairy, cereal bars and biscuits. Can replace with buckwheat or rice cakes with nut butters.

Treatment

Repeat all previous prescriptions:
Rx.1, Rx.2, Rx.3, Rx.4

Added in

Rx.5 External use

Artemisia dracunculus EO	2 ml
Chamomila recutita EO	1 ml
Lavandula angustifolia EO	3 ml
Calendula officinalis macerated oil	100 ml

Sig: apply lotion to the sternum, solar plexus and epigastric region bid

Rationale for prescription

Artemisia EO as a splanchnic decongestant and to reduce parasympathetic activity. *Chamomila* EO to reduce parasympathetic and alphasympathetic activity. *Lavandula* EO to reduce alphasympathetic activity.

Follow-up appointment 1 month later

- Reduced bloating after eating. Last few days, however, the gut has been 'churning' a lot again. Feels that he bloats more when cold.
- Patient reports losing weight, but this is a good thing he feels. The patient feels like the 'strange symptoms' he described previously are going now.
- Pain in groin fluctuated for about 4 days, but has now gone.
- Reports improvement in energy; no longer napping in afternoons, but energy is still not optimal and effected by the winter.
- A couple of days following sex, experiences some pain in the chest and dizziness.
- Reports experiencing pain on the left side of the chest last week.
- Some pain in sternum; feels related to reflux. Patient reports it relaxes and improves when he presses it. Used omeprazole just once since the last appointment.
- Experiencing some neck pain and stiffness.

Diet

- Has stopped all dairy, sugar and cereal bars
- Eating steak and roast potatoes for dinner
- Using almond butter
- 2–3 bananas daily
- Has started eating dried fruits

GIT

- No flatulence
- Some bloating, reports increased with cold weather

Findings

- Tongue not as white now.

Advice

Avoid dried fruits containing sulphur as it can cause bloating and irritation.

Treatment

Repeat Rx.1, Rx.2

Rx.3

Agrimonia eupatoria	15 ml
Gentiana lutea	10 ml
Centaurium erythraea	15 ml
Passiflora incarnata	20 ml
Withania somnifera	25 ml
Ribes nigrum	20 ml
Sig: 5 ml tid	

Rationale for prescription

Agrimonia to support pancreatic activity and reduces parasympathetic activity indirectly by its effect on the pancreas. *Gentiana* and *Centaurium* for the effects already mentioned. *Passiflora* to reduce alphasympathetic activity. *Withania* as a tonic herb to assist in energy and stamina. As a bitter, it aids in digestion. *Ribes* to support adrenals. The patient says his energy is affected in the winter, so it is important to support the adrenal glands at this time.

Rx.4

Probiotic as before

Rx.5

Digestive enzyme—recommended Biocare bioenzyme; Sig: 1 od to begin with and see how it is tolerated. Only to be taken with food.

This is to support the pancreas. Enzymes can be a very effective part of the treatment, and again by supporting the pancreas can assist in reducing parasympathetic activity.

Follow-up appointment 5 weeks later

- Pain in back and pain in the abdomen (lower right side) has gone and is fine now.
- Every time has sex and ejaculates, the next day gets pain in the central region of solar plexus and also gets cough; it usually lasts about 2 days. Pain is generally better, no more pain in muscles and joints like before.
- Energy is good, much better. Feels that in the past had no energy unless took omeprazole.
- The patient feels he is now coping better with stress.
- Patient reports hands and legs get very cold.
- Not using omeprazole, only after sex when symptoms return.
- Developed rash on the left side of the groin with a strong odour. Using Canesten cream which helps. Some itching on right foot only.
- Has to desire to have sex; however, difficulty getting fully erect; reports has been like this for years. Sometimes takes Viagra. Feels strongly that past contraction of gonorrhoea is affecting him.

Took digestive enzymes for 1 day at a dose of 1 tid instead of what was advised (1 od). Experienced lots of loose stools the next day and ceased taking them.

Diet

- Maintained no diary
- One coffee daily, sometimes none, with ½ teaspoon sugar
- No other sugar
- No bread

GIT

- No more bloating

Findings

- Tongue no longer white-coated

Treatment

Repeat prescriptions Rx.1, Rx.2

Rx.3

Agrimonia eupatoria	15 ml
Gentiana lutea	10 ml
Passiflora incarnata	20 ml
Withania somnifera	25 ml
Ribes nigrum GM	30 ml
Rhodiola Rosea	20 ml

Sig: 8.5 ml bid

Rationale for prescription

Added *Rhodiola* simply as an adaptogen for its regulating effects.

Rx.4

Probiotic as before

Rx.5

Glycyrrhiza glabra decoction to be used specifically after intercourse
Sig: 1 tsp as decoction tid
To support adrenals more, specifically after ejaculation. When a male ejaculates there is a large beta discharge which can deplete the adrenals even more. This causes a disturbance in the autonomic nervous system, i.e. effecting the LES; hence the pain in the solar plexus.

Follow-up appointment 1 month later

- Patient reports that pain in abdomen and back remains okay.
- Has completely ceased use of omeprazole.
- Feels that digestion is good now.
- No longer feels tired; has good energy levels and much more stamina.
- No more pain in the solar plexus region.
- Rash in the groin area, left side comes and goes but is overall better, and odour has gone. Feet are no longer itching.
- Patient reports he feels calmer and is coping okay with stress.
- Reports that erectile difficulty is fine now with no problems.

Did not take Rx.5 due to it being out of stock at the time of the consultation and did not come back to purchase it. Reports that cough can come back after sex and last a couple of weeks.

Diet

- Very good, but has started eating cereal and cake
- Has coffee only rarely; no longer every day

GIT

- No bloating
- Opens bowel daily, no problems
- Feels has been improving incrementally by 20% every month

Findings

- Splanchnic congestion still high ++++
- Some tenderness in the colon and in the ileocecal region

Treatment

Advised to use buckwheat flour to make pancakes as an alternative to conventional pancakes.
Repeat prescriptions Rx.1, Rx.2, Rx.3

Rx.4

Probiotics: try a different brand in order to vary probiotic strains

Rx.5

Solgar curcumin ()
Sig: 1 bid
As an anti-inflammatory to assist in inflammation of the bowel. The *Solgar curcumin* is in liquid form, in a soft gel and it is in a form that seems very gentle on the stomach. I use this brand for patients with sensitive stomachs.

Rx. 6

Glycyrrhiza glabra decoction to be used specifically after intercourse
Sig: 1 tsp as decoction tid
The patient took this prescription a while longer and then ceased as he was happy with where he was health-wise.

Case 6

A 4-year-old male presenting with constipation, which started April last year. Developed a fissure. Before that, had no problems opening bowels. Fissure developed, followed by severe constipation. Has gone up to 12 days without opening bowels. Has to use nappies as is scared of using the toilet.

Last January, mother returned to work, and the child did not respond well to this. This was demonstrated by a change in his behaviour, which became more challenging, then returned to normal around April time. Mother reports that the child has a good imagination.

X-ray in Columbia revealed impacted faeces, which was treated with enemas. Also treated with laxatives.

Mother reports no major problems during pregnancy or birth, but it was a forceps delivery. Low weight and low blood sugar but not premature. Breastfed for 6 months, then after a combination of breastfeeding and food until 14 months. Has a good immunity with no infections so far.

Plays and interacts well with other children; plays tennis, football and swims.

Sleep

- Wakes 2–3 times a night. On a good night will only wake twice.
- Has never slept well.
- Sometimes has bad dreams. He is afraid of monsters and big dogs. Not rested in the mornings.
- Using homoeopathic remedies for sleep.

Diet

- Used to have a lot of dairy, but has cut this down by 90%
- Lots of fruit and vegetables, 5–6 portions of fruit daily
- Cutting down on pasta and rice
- Uses only oil on salads
- No takeaways
- Fibre-rich cereals with goat's milk for breakfast

Findings

- Little adrenal congestion ++
- Distended abdomen
- Splanchnic region: Little liver and pancreas congestion ++
- Eyelids tremble a little when closed ++
- Glabellar tap; blink response rapid +++
- No record of the temperature of hands and feet

Advice

Avoid gluten, dairy and sugar. Avoid bananas.

Explaining the case

From birth, there was an aggression on the organism with regards to the forceps delivery. The aggression stimulated the alphasympathetic system. There could have been more complex issues with the pregnancy that we are unaware of. Sometimes the information is not disclosed for whatever reason, or simply forgotten. In addition to this, the fistula is another form of aggression, physically and psychologically. The pain resulted in a fear of passing stools. The child was further stressed by the fact that in January, his mother went back to work. This was a substantial change for the child, as his environment altered. These factors would have all stimulated alphasympathetic activity.

As alpha increases, there is a reduction in gastrointestinal motility as alpha is a constrictive system. In addition to this, the child would have been consciously holding onto his stools for fear of pain when opening his bowels. The adrenals are implicated, as they are involved in the adaptation phenomenon. They are needed for the organism to correctly adapt to aggression. Remember that betasympathetic activity is the release mechanism; needed to relax the anal sphincter for bowel evacuation to occur.

It is likely that TRH is involved due to the various types of aggression that occurred. Waking several times through the night and the restless sleep can be linked to high central alpha (dopamine) and high central beta (TRH). With the bad dreams being linked to the elevated TRH. Parasympathetic activity rises at night in order to induce sleep. Alphasympathetic activity also rises but is lower than para. When alpha breaks through (rises above para) then waking occurs. Beta follows alpha in the cycle, and beta brings with it the activity.

In addition to all of this, we must not forget the toxicity element. Toxins are forms of aggression on the organism. The constipation will cause a toxic overload as the toxins generated from metabolism will not be excreted efficiently and i.e. reabsorbed into the system. Constipation and intestinal congestion, will cause a modification in the microbiome. As we have seen in previous chapters, the microbiome of the gut has far-reaching effects well beyond the bowel. This can affect the activity of the brain.

Treatment plan

- The main part of the treatment is to reduce alphasympathetic activity.
- Support adrenals.
- Reduce TRH.
- Cleanse colon.
- Provide a laxative effect.
- Mechanical stimulation of bowel.

Treatment

Rx. 1

Lotion for abdominal massage
Rosemarinus officinalis EO   15 gtt

Lavandula angustifolia EO	1 ml
Chamomilla recutita EO	10 gtt
Calendula officinalis macerated oil	100 ml

Sig: massage into the abdomen for 5 minutes, tid, in a clockwise motion

Rationale for prescription

Providing a lotion which is to be massaged onto the abdomen is a very useful part of the treatment in such cases. It will allow the child some much-needed time for affection from his mother, thus helping him on a psychological and physiological level. In addition to this, there will be therapeutic benefits from the essential oils in the lotion. It is very important that the person performing the massage, in this case the mother, be calm and relaxed when performing the massage, as it will be felt by the child as well as transmitted through the hands.

Lavandula was used for its superb alphasympatholytic properties as well as its ability to relax the sphincter of Oddi, thus improving motility. *Rosmarinus* for its warming and circulatory stimulating properties and to assist in liver drainage. *Chamomilla* as an antispasmodic and alphasympatholytic. Remember if essential oils are used frequently enough, they will absorb through the skin and have a systemic effect. *Calendula* as a base oil but you could just as easily use olive oil or any other suitable base oil. It is very important to massage in a clockwise motion following the natural flow of elimination.

Rx.2

Magnesium (recommend Biocare bio-magnesium)
Sig: 1 od; open capsule and mix powder in some water
To relax the bowel and support the nervous system.

Rx.3

Flaxseed oil and olive oil
Sig: 1 tsp of each daily, first thing in the morning with a small cup of warm water
As a natural laxative.

Rx.4

Lavandula angustifolia	15 ml
Leonurus cardiaca	10 ml
Melissa officinalis	10 ml
Passiflora incarnata	10 ml
Glycyrrhiza glabra 1:1	10 ml

Sig: 40 gtt tid

Rationale for prescription

Lavandula and *Passiflora* for their alphasympatholytic effects. *Leonurus* to reduce TRH activity. *Melissa* to reduce alphasympathetic activity, and this is another plant that is effective at relaxing the sphincter of Oddi, thus assisting in drainage. *Glycyrrhiza* to support the adrenal glands and for its useful laxative action.

Follow-up appointment 1 month later

- Mother reports the child has been complaining of stomach ache after opening bowels, but it does not last long.
- Massage is going well, and the child likes it. Performing massage 2–3 times daily.
- Couldn't use the bio-magnesium as did not like the taste. Used magnesium oxide 350 mg instead and gave ½ once daily, but only for 5 days. Had this at home.
- Using homoeopathic remedies recommended by homoeopath: *chamomilla, gelsemium, kalmia, stramonium*. Helps a little.
- Has only been giving 20 gtt of the tincture tid as the child doesn't want to drink it due to the taste. Giving it in juice helps.

Sleep

- Waking at night still, moves a lot through the night and not relaxing
- Often tired next day
- Some nights does not sleep

GIT

- Has improved a lot since the initial consultation.
- Day after the first consult, opened bowels while sleeping, and this happened a few times (see Table 27).

Table 27.

Day	Opened bowels	Location
Thursday	Yes	Once, whilst sleeping
Friday	Yes	Once, whilst sleeping
Saturday	No	
Sunday	No	
Monday	No	
Tuesday	Yes	Once, whilst sleeping
Wednesday	Yes	Twice, on toilet and whilst sleeping

(*Continued*)

Table 27. (Continued)

Day	Opened bowels	Location
Thursday	Yes	Twice, on toilet and whilst sleeping
Friday	Yes	Once, whilst sleeping
Saturday	Yes	Once, on toilet
Sunday	No	
Monday	Yes	Once, on toilet

Findings

- The abdomen was much better; not as distended, softer but a bit tender.
- Warm, dry hands and not damp.

Treatment

Repeat Rx.1 and Rx.3 as before

Rx.2

Magnesium oxide (as has this at home already)
Use the same dose as before for a few days at a time
Repeat Rx.4
Sig: continue with 20 gtt tid and try to increase to 40 gtt tid

Rx.5

Optibac Probiotics for constipation
Sig: ½ sachet daily
This probiotic has probiotic strains mixed with fibre to assist in constipation.

Follow-up appointment 3 weeks later

- Has been able to increase tincture to 30 gtt tid and trying to build up to 40 gtt. Used laxatives once since the last appointment.
- Taking oils in the morning as recommended.
- Mother feels the probiotic used did not help.
- Childs abdomen is now swollen and so he does not like to have it massaged. It is possible that the bowel is sensitive to the fibre in the probiotic.
- Last 2 days he's been very distressed; shouting for no understandable reason and having lots of tantrums.

GIT

- Has opened bowels only five times in the last 3 weeks
- Twice while sleeping and three times whilst awake
- Having stomach aches every now and again

Sleep

- Same as before

Treatment

Repeat Rx.1, Rx.2 and Rx.3
Stop probiotic for constipation
Also added in fish oil as a source of Omega 3

Rx.4

Lavandula angustifolia	15 ml
Taraxacum officinale Radix	10 ml
Carduus marianus	10 ml
Melissa officinalis	10 ml
Passiflora incarnata	10 ml
Glycyrrhiza glabra 1:1	10 ml
Sig: 40 gtt tid increase slowly	

Rationale for prescription

Removed *Leonorus* (not enough space in prescription), as felt there were enough sympatholytic plants to assist indirectly in reducing TRH by decreasing alpha, and it was necessary to drain the liver at this stage. Added in *Taraxacum* and *Carduus* in order to drain the liver.

Rx.5

Ribes nigrum	50 ml

Sig: 30 gtt bid
To support adrenals. This will further assist in rebalancing the autonomic nervous system.

Follow-up appointment 3 weeks later

- Has been taking the full dose of the tincture with no problems.

- Things are improving again. The first week after the last consultation, opened bowels three times in the week whilst sleeping. The second week, five times whilst awake. The third week, five times whilst aware and has been sitting on the toilet. The child was a bit anxious in the beginning about using the toilet but now does so with no problem. In the past 2 weeks has stopped using nappies.
- Mum reports that she feels things got worse when continuing with magnesium oxide so stopped and felt things seemed to get better. Could be a coincidence.

Sleep

- Falls asleep okay but wakes often and can sometimes come to mum's bed.
- No bad dreams like previously.
- In the morning, while sleeping, asks for food, pancakes, eggs, etc.

GIT

- Stomach not really hurting now; the child says it does a bit during tummy massage.
- Appetite has increased.
- Can have a lot of flatulence, not smelly, mostly in the morning.

Findings

- Skin a bit dry; some bumps on the stomach. Advised to use coconut oil on the area.
- No pancreatic congestion or liver congestion.
- The abdomen is soft now.
- Adrenals a bit congested ++.
- Hands and feet a bit sticky.

Treatment

Stop Rx.2 (magnesium)
Repeat Rx.1, Rx.3, Rx.4, Rx.5
Carry on with fish oil

Rx.6

Leonurus cardiaca	10 ml
Lavandula angustifolia	10 ml
Tilia europaea	10 ml
Citrus aurantium flos	10 ml
Passiflora incarnata	10 ml

Sig: 15–20 gtt noct od
For sleep to reduce alphasympathetic activity and TRH levels at night.

Follow-up appointment 1 month later

- Has been exercising in a lot in the past few weeks; more tennis, swimming and other sports.
- Mother has noticed that mood is good and no tantrums like previously. Does get very upset when he can't open his bowels though. This happens only when he is on the toilet and is constipated.
- Has been taking all medications as directed.

Sleep

- Sleeping a lot better with the sleeping formula.
- Not waking up as much or as early now.
- Still moves a lot when asleep, can end up on the floor but then gets back into bed.

GIT

- Bowel habits: a bit more constipated than before.
- Mother has not been compliant with the diet advice.

Findings

- Abdomen not distended much, but there was some fullness in the ileocecal region.
- White tongue.

Treatment

Repeat Rx.1, Rx.3, Rx4, Rx.5, Rx.6
Carry on with fish oil

Rx.7

Saccharomyces boulardii (probiotic) for children
Sig: 1 sachet BD
As an anti-fungal.

Rx.8

Optibac Children's Probiotic
Sig: ½ to 1 sachet a day
To assist in rebalancing the microbiome of the gut.

Rx.9

> Reintroduce magnesium again for a while
> Sig: ½ tablet od
> To assist with constipation.

Advice

Very important to be compliant with the diet. Strictly no:

- Gluten, sugar or dairy at all for 1 month to see how he responds
- See osteopath for examination

Follow-up appointment 1 month later

The patient has been doing very well. Opening his bowels more often, but parents have to remind him to open his bowels as he does not feel the urge to do so himself. Responds well with a reminder.

His mother reports that he continues to have tantrums for no obvious reason. For example, if he writes a letter and then his mother suggests to write a word in a particular way, he becomes very upset and emotional.

Continues to keep up a lot of sports and physical activity (tennis, swimming, etc.).

While in Egypt on holiday the previous month, he was opening his bowels every 2 days; parents could notice that he was resisting and 'holding it in'. When they returned at the end of the month, he began opening his bowels daily and has not passed a stool whilst sleeping.

They have established an evening routine, and it appears to be helping (toilet, bath, bed). Advised to give water after baths as can be dehydrating. He has started psychotherapy; the therapist is aware of current herbal treatments.

He is starting to get 'bored' of the abdominal massage.

Sleep

- Sleep is good when sleep drops are used. Parents sometimes forget to administer them and notice disturbed sleep or not sleeping through the night.

GIT

- Opening bowels nearly every day now
- Good appetite

Diet

- On a low sugar diet
- No dairy, with the exception of some yoghurt given at school

Treatment

Repeat all medication as before.

Follow-up appointment 5 weeks later

Treatment is going well. Continued averaging bowel movements every other day, except for the last 4 days, when he has been opening his bowels daily. Ran out of medicine for 2 days, and on these days the child panicked and cried and did not want to sit on the toilet. Otherwise responds well to being prompted to use the toilet; he is still not initiating this himself as he still doesn't seem to 'feel' it. On one occasion, he used the toilet without prompting.

Tantrums are not as bad now. Going well with the psychologist. Using praise techniques. Parents have been trying to change his toilet habits to morning and lunch, instead of evenings. Has not opened bowels whilst sleeping. Good sleep quality over the last few weeks, only waking on some occasions, but falls back to sleep straight away. He has been biting his nails and fingertips.

Diet

- Has been eating ice cream (i.e. dairy and sugar) as it's summertime
- Decreased appetite; possibly due to the heat
- Has been drinking less water but managing some water after baths to promote hydration

Findings

- Much less congestion in the splanchnic region
- No adrenal congestion
- White patches on the tongue

Treatment

Advised: No ice cream and cut out sugar completely, including fruit.
Repeat all medication as before but made a change to Rx.4.

Rx.4

Olea europaea	10 ml
Lavandula angustifolia	15 ml
Taraxacum officinale Radix	10 ml
Carduus marianus	10 ml
Passiflora incarnata	10 ml
Glycyrrhiza glabra 1:1	10 ml
Sig: 40 gtt tid	

Rationale for prescription

Added *Olea* as an anti-fungal plant.

Follow-up appointment 6 weeks later

Developed a cough a few weeks ago that lasted approx. 4 days. Thick green mucus for 3 days. Used a pharmacy cough medicine for 2 days.

Tantrums are a lot better now., but he is still biting his fingernails and fingertips.

GIT

- Opened bowels every day for 2 weeks. Missed 2 days while on holiday. Improvement from every other day.
- Now occasionally going to the toilet on his own, without prompting. Parents have been giving lots of praise and encouragement for this.

Diet

- Not going well with diet. Difficulty stopping sweets (juice, biscuits)
- Tried for 1 week, but the child became very upset by this
- Have reduced ice cream but not cut it out
- Having goat's cheese, but no cow products

Sleep

- Stopped the sleep medicine as it ran out
- Sleep has improved and sleeping through the whole night 2–3 nights per week

Treatment

Repeat all medication as before but made a change to Rx.5.

Rx.4

Olea europaea	10 ml
Lavandula angustifolia	15 ml
Taraxacum officinale Radix	10 ml
Carduus marianus	10 ml
Passiflora incarnata	10 ml
Leonorus cardiaca	10 ml

Sig: 40 gtt tid

Rationale for prescription

Removed *Glycyrrhiza* as the patient has been taking it for quite some time. Added in *Leonorus* to assist in reducing TRH in the day time. The biting of the nails and finger-tips is an obsessive behaviour and linked to high TRH activity. Dopamine (central alpha) is also most linked to this behaviour.

Follow-up appointment 2 months later

Cough cleared up. Doing very well.

He has stopped biting his fingers and nails. Last week mother cut his growing fingernails for the first time. He is more frequently going to the toilet by himself and even when out he has been able to go to the toilet. So much better. A little prompting needed on some occasions.

He is having some pain in the legs and knees. Likely growing pains, happening more in mornings and evenings.

GIT

- September: opened bowels every day except 5 days throughout the month
- October, every day, except 3 days in total
- No stomach aches at all

Diet

- Giving lots of fibre
- Using almond milk; no dairy
- Sugar/sweets only twice a week as a treat

Sleep

- Very good now; sleeping all night, in his own bed

Treatment

- Stop *Saccharomyces boulardii* (probiotic)
- Stop Ribes nigrum
- Carry on flaxseed oil and olive oil + fish oil
- Carry on Optibac probiotic for children
- Carry on magnesium; Sig: ½ tablet od
- Use Biocare multivitamin powder
- Carry on Rx.4

Follow-up appointment 2.5 months later

- Overall, doing very well.
- Continues not to bite nails. Developed a slight cough and recovered very quickly.
- Pain in legs and knees much better.

GIT

- Opens bowels every day now.
- Went every day but 2 days last month; this was a very busy period for him (birthday), lots of meet-ups and dates with friends, etc.
- Working on using toilet outside of the house, as he is not keen on this.
- No stomach aches.

Diet

- Added in banana and no problems noticed. Having one, 1–2 times a week
- Diet good otherwise

Sleep

- Sometimes wakes once in the night; goes to his mother's bed, but then goes back to his own bed after directed by his mother to return

Treatment

- As the patient was doing so well, advised to wean off medication and see how he responds.
- Reduce main formula Rx.4 by half for 3 weeks, then half again for 3 weeks, then stop.
- Decrease magnesium, Sig: 1/3 tablet od; stop in 3–6 weeks.
- Stop flax oil.
- Advised to use fish oil, probiotics and vitamins cycling on and off.

Case 7

A 51-year-old female, presenting with Crohn's and celiac disease. Developed hyperthyroidism 15–20 years ago and was very unwell. Prescribed Carbimazole, but it was ineffective. Underwent radioactive iodine therapy that killed off the thyroid and was not put onto thyroxin and nearly died. Commenced thyroxin and things started to improve and felt good.

Sometime after, developed digestive symptoms and experienced light bleeding for 2–3 years. Was eventually diagnosed with Crohn's disease. During the same period, the patient also discovered she had celiac disease.

Underwent three colonoscopies in 2010, which found mild inflammation at the ileo-cecal junction, very first part (right at the start) of the ascending colon and in the transverse colon (slightly off centre towards the right side). Active inflammation found in the rectum. Endoscopy also; diagnosed gastritis. These sights were marked out on a diagram from the report of the colonoscopy that the patient brought to the clinic.

Prescribed prednisolone but developed side effects of hallucinations, sleep disturbance and dizziness.

The patient feels like she is in a state of permanent 'flare-up' of her Crohn's. Regular bleeding from bowel/rectum (red blood) and can experience increased bleeding with clots when flare-up state worsens.

Other symptoms include watery eyes, that can sometimes weep for weeks, red eyes and 'raw' lips, also for weeks at a time.

Stopped smoking 3 years ago. Consumes occasional alcohol (spirits/gin).

Past

- Had keyhole surgery on left knee.
- Grandfather died 21 years ago; she had an infant at the time and believes her breast milk dried up due to the severity of stress.
- Severe allergy to some tropical fruits (melon, passion fruit, pineapple, etc.). Has experienced anaphylactic shock and carries an EpiPen.

Medications

- Thyroxin   100 micrograms od
- Cetirizine   10 mg od
- Azathioprine   75 mg
- Balsalazide   patient can't remember the dosage

Other supplements

- Chamomile tea (finds helpful)
- Glucosamine and chondroitin
- Vitamin C 1000 mg od
- B12 capsules
- Probiotics VSL 3

Family history

N/A

GIT

- Opens bowels very often; at worst every 20 minutes, with bleeding every time

- Despite high pain threshold, feels she has severe pain in the bowels (e.g. underwent root canal without analgesia). Pain so severe that sometimes feels like could pass out
- No mucous and no undigested food in stools

Sleep

- Generally, very tired
- Falls asleep easily, wakes three times a night to open bowels

Findings

- Cold feet and cold hands +++
- Damp feet and hands +
- Pancreatic congestion ++++
- Slight liver congestion +
- Adrenal congestion +++++
- Delayed and prolonged skin redness ++++
- White tongue +++
- Some white patches on nails

Explaining the case

It is evident from the clinical examination and case history that there is high para- and alphasympathetic activity. The hands are not very damp, but there is a substantial amount of pancreatic congestion present. The increased gut motility is also linked to a high parasympathetic state. It is very important to address the pancreatic congestion in Crohn's disease. The redness of the skin is linked to high histamine as a result of the high alpha and adrenal issues. White patches on nails are usually as a result of zinc deficiency. Once the mucosa heals, and the patient starts to digest and absorb nutrients properly, this usually clears. It may be useful to supplement with zinc also.

This patient does not have a working thyroid gland and so has to take thyroxin. Thyroxin can induce a state of inflammation. As I have seen in nearly all my patients on thyroxin; when looking at the functional biology results, the thyroid metabolic, insulin, free radical and inflammation indexes are very commonly elevated. It is not a simple task to get the dose of thyroxin right, especially from just looking at TSH levels. Most patients are found to be overmedicated, and this has very negative metabolic effects. The functional biology helps tremendously in evaluating this metabolic disturbance and helps in getting the dose of thyroxin right in patients that do not have a functioning thyroid. As we have looked at previously, insulin is a cause of tissular inflammation and increases free radical activity. This was undoubtedly a factor in the development of Crohn's disease. We have no information as to whether or not there was an autoimmune thyroid condition present in the past as the patient did not have any information with her.

Colonoscopy revealed inflammation in the rectum, ileocecal region and transverse colon (slightly off centre to the right side). These sights are related to the receptors ACTH and FSH. Please see Figure 18, Chapter 12.

Treatment plan

- Reduce para and alpha
- Reduce FSH activity
- Support adrenal glands and sustain peripheral beta activity
- Drain and support pancreas
- Reduce spasm
- Reduce inflammation
- Restore microbiome

There are most likely other pathways that need addressing, but we do not have a functional biology to work with. It would be very useful to look at the thyroid indexes, insulin index and free radical indexes, from the functional biology to assess what effect the thyroxin is having on the patient.

Treatment

Rx. 1

Chamomillla recutita infusion
Sig: 3 tsp per infusion tid
To reduce para- and alphasympathetic activity, as an anti-inflammatory and antispasmodic.

Rx.2

Can continue B12 capsules as before

Rx.3

Lithospermum officinale	10 ml
Vitex agnus-castus	7 ml
Chamomilla recutita	20 ml
Viburnum opulus	20 ml
Glycyrrhiza glabra 1:3	20 ml
Artemisia absinthium	5 ml
Astragalus membranaceus	20 ml
Sig: 5–7.5 ml bid	

Rationale for prescription

Lithospermum and *Vitex* to reduce FSH activity. *Chamomilla* to reduce alpha and para-sympathetic activity, as an anti-inflammatory and antispasmodic. *Viburnum* as an antispasmodic and alphasympatholytic. *Glycyrrhiza* to support adrenals and peripheral beta activity. *Artemisia* as an anti-fungal, bitter to support digestion and anti-inflammatory. Research shows that *Artemisia* accelerates the healing process in Cohn's patients. It possesses a steroid-sparing effect.[227,228] Astragalus as a tonic herb to help with low energy. It also has anti-inflammatory and antioxidant properties and has a specific use in the treating of inflamed intestinal epithelial cells, according to research in 2018.[229]

Rx.4

Curcumin
Sig: 1 bid
As an anti-inflammatory.

Rx.5

Green Clay
Sig: 1 tsp bid soaked in a glass of water and consumed ½ hour before breakfast and before bed
As an anti-inflammatory and anti-ulcer, green clay is very effective at stopping gastrointestinal bleeding.

Rx.6

Carry on taking probiotics
To help treat dysbiosis.

Advice

Follow gluten-free, daily free, sugar-free, yeast-free and caffeine-free diet. Only consume the following vegetables to begin with: carrot, green beans without strings, pumpkin, butternut squash, broccoli heads (no stalks). These vegetables must be cooked very well so that they are soft. No spicy food. Fish and meat cooked plainly as soup or roast. Some white potato or white rice is allowed. No brown rice as the fibre in brown rice is extremely irritating. No fruit and no fruit juice.

At this time, I had not been trained as a GAPS practitioner. If I had been, I would have recommended the GAPS protocol.

Follow-up appointment 1 month later

- The first week following the last appointment, bleeding near enough ceased.
- The severity of pain has also improved following the first week.
- On 6th or 7th night, the patient had a gin and tonic and experienced diarrhoea the next day; felt better the day after that. Bleeding started again following this.
- Feeling worried as son travelling to the Middle East. Has also been feeling angry at times.
- Reduced balsalazide dose from 6 to 3, of her own accord. Initially stopped but noticed the return of some bleeding, so increased dose back up to 3.
- Stopped azathioprine, of her own accord, after gradual reduction. Did not notice any difference other than the return of a croaky voice, which was present during the initial stages of diagnosis.
- Generally feeling better. Energy not as bad as before. The patient feels that there may be an issue with her thyroid medication and needs to have it checked.
- Soreness on lips has improved considerably. The skin has also improved. Lips started swelling 2 days ago after introducing fruit juice back into diet. Advised patient to stop this as could be causing problems for her.

Diet

- Has been sticking regularly to the diet sheet provided; cut out tea and coffee, drinking only herbal teas
- Tried eating prawns but stopped as felt might be related to return of bleeding
- Lost 6 lb in the first week, gained 2 lb in the second week and the weight seems stable now
- Having 100% puffed rice with rice milk for breakfast

GIT

- Having some flatulence, only when passing blood and mostly in the morning.
- Big improvement in frequency of opening bowels:
  - The first week opened bowels approx. ten times a day
  - Now approx. five times a day
- Can notice some red bleeding when opening bowels at night, however, has reduced a lot since starting treatment.
- Some pain but the patient feels it is due to flatulence.

Sleep

- Not often waking at night to open bowels

Treatment

Continue with dietary advice.

Repeat

- Green clay
- *Chamomilla* infusion
- *Curcumin*
- B12 capsule
- Probiotics

Added in

Activated charcoal
Sig: follow dose on the package
To help with flatulence.

Rx.3

Agrimonia eupatoria	15 ml
Vitex agnus-castus	7 ml
Lithospermum officinale	15 ml
Chamomilla recutita	20 ml
Hydrastis canadensis	20 ml
Glycyrrhiza glabra 1:3	15 ml
Artemisia absinthium	5 ml
Viburnum opulus	5 ml

Sig: 7.5 ml bid

Rationale for prescription

Removed Astragalus and reduced the dose of Viburnum in order to make space for *Hydrastis* and *Agrimonia*. *Hydrastis* is very effective as an anti-inflammatory, mucous membrane restorative and astringent assisting in stopping the bleeding. Added *Agrimonia*, as a pancreatic drainer, reduces parasympathetic activity indirectly by supporting pancreas, is also anti-inflammatory.

Follow-up appointment 1 month later

- Generally feeling well. Experienced a flare-up 2 days ago as had some cake.
- Has stopped all allopathic medications for Crohn's. Reports that charcoal helps a lot.

- A cream recommended by GP has helped a lot with swelling and itching lips and neck.
- Is now exercising 1 hour a day.

Medications

- Thyroxin
- Cetirizine

Diet

- Eating more variety of foods; increased amount of vegetables
- Still no refined sugar
- Not eating any junk food
- Eating more fish and meat
- Having some cheese now

GIT

- Opening bowels approximately seven times a daily
- Some blood loss in the morning, but not much
- Not waking at night to open bowels

Findings

- Adrenal congestion +++++
- Prolonged skin redness +++
- Pancreatic congestion ++
- Cold feet and cold hands ++
- Damp feet and hands +
- White tongue ++

Improvements

Hands are a little warmer, slightly less skin redness and pancreatic congestion much improved.

Advice

Add in new foods on a 3-day cycle, e.g. eggs. Stay off all refined sugar, gluten, caffeine, yeast, milk and all processed food.

Treatment

Repeat

- Green clay
- *Curcumin*
- Probiotic
- Activated charcoal
- *Chamomilla* infusion
- Rx.3

Added in Lamberts L-glutamine capsules 500 mg
Sig: 2 capsules bid, then after 1 week increase to 3 capsules bid
To assist in repair of the gastrointestinal mucosa.

Follow-up appointment 1 month later (brief, by phone)

Called and said experienced bad histamine reaction and had to go to the hospital. Anaphylaxis last Monday. Prescribed prednisolone 40 mg for 5 days.

Prescribed

- Vitamin C—sig: 1000 mg qid
- Lambert's quercetin—sig: 500 mg 1 od

To reduce histamine.

Follow-up appointment 3 weeks later

- Patient reports that allergy response has settled down. Completed 5 days of prednisolone and carried on with the quercetin and vitamin C and no further allergic episodes since and no swelling of lips.
- Experienced some constipation, so reduced clay as recommended to once daily and now things are fine.
- Still not using any allopathic medications for Crohn's.
- Has been exercising every other day and has lost a couple of dress sizes.
- Blood pressure: 102/82.

Diet

- Using gluten-free bread, dairy-free spread, no coffee
- Some tea, feels okay with it
- Odd bit of milk and cheese once a week
- No refined sugar, no cakes, biscuits, chocolate, etc.

- Has added in eggs, baked beans, mushrooms
- Allergic to nuts

GIT

- Opening bowels 1–2 times daily, very good improvement.
- Still feels some discomfort and spasmodic pain, only when needing to pass stools, otherwise feels well.
- No blood at all in stools.
- Some flatulence; sometimes smelly.
- White patches in nails have gone.

Advised not to consume milk.

Treatment

Carry on with all supplements as before
Advised to switch from L-glutamine capsules to the powder to enable ease of increasing dose
Sig: 5 grams od/bid

Rx.3

Plantago major	5 ml
Chamomilla recutita	20 ml
Glycyrrhiza glabra 1:3	15 ml
Andrographis paniculata	20 ml
Agrimonia eupatoria	15 ml
Artemisia absinthium	5 ml
Vitex agnus-castus	7 ml
Viburnum opulus	5 ml
Rehmannia glutinosa prepared root	10 ml
Sig: 7.5 ml bd	

Rationale for prescription

Removed *Hydrastis*. Break from *Hydrastis* and replaced with Andrographis. *Andrographis* is another useful anti-inflammatory plant. *Lithospermum* was out of stock so added *Rehmannia* to support the adrenals more in light of the allergic issues. Added *Plantago* as well. Plantago is an anti-allergic plant but also a valuable intestinal drainer. *Rehmannia* and *Plantago* do not replace the effect of *Lithospermum* as *Lithospermum* is used to reduce gonadotropins, but they have other useful actions as mentioned. The *Lithospermum* will be reintroduced once back in stock.

Follow-up appointment 6 weeks later

- Patient reports approximate loss of 1.5 stone in the last 3 weeks (was 12.6 stone; now 11.2 stone). Attributes this to the recent stress of parents getting divorced and having to attend court. In the 24 hours before the court date, the patient lost 3 lbs. Weight has stabilised since the stress of court has come to an end.
- No episodes of facial swelling; lip-tingling on a couple of occasions but no allergic reactions.
- Has recently stopped exercising.
- Blood pressure: 130/90—is under stress.

Medications

- Thyroxin 100 micrograms
- Cetirizine 1 od

Diet

- Not recently eating much due to stress

GIT

- No bleeding at all
- No diarrhoea, no mucus
- Opening bowels once a day or every other day
- Not experiencing bloating in stomach after eating

Findings

- Adrenal congestion ++++
- Pancreatic congestion ++
- Generalised tenderness, especially in the ileocecal region
- Cold feet and hands +
- Damp hands and feet +

Treatment

Repeat all supplements that was previously taking.

Added in

Biohealth passiflora capsules
Sig: 2 tid

In order to reduce alphasympathetic activity in light of the extra stress, she has been under.

Rx.3

Agrimonia eupatoria	15 ml
Vitex agnus-castus	7 ml
Lithospermum officinale	15 ml
Hydrastis canadensis	20 ml
Chamomilla recutita	20 ml
Glycyrrhiza glabra 1:3	15 ml
Artemisia absinthium	5 ml
Viburnum opulus	5 ml
Sig: 7.5 ml bid	

Rationale for prescription

Added *Lithospernmum* back in as it was back in stock. As the patient had a break from *Hydrastis*, I added it back into the formula.

Follow-up appointment 1 month later

- Blood test results back from GP from a few weeks ago. TSH about 7. Patient reports GP confused as TSH is up so would indicate needs more thyroxin, however, is losing weight not gaining weight, which should be the case in a hypothyroid state. GP will retest in 1 month before altering the dose of the thyroxin.
- Family problems are ongoing; however, less stressful. Lost about 1.5 stone in weight. Now 11 stone.
- Working extended hours, however, work is enjoyable and not stressful.
- Lips dry and sore on occasion, but no pain/tingling or allergic responses.
- Energy is okay. Not currently exercising.
- Blood pressure: 95/70.

GIT

- Appetite not great, eating small meals
- Feels full easily; can go all day with no food
- No blood in stools; some diarrhoea
- Opening bowels 3–4 times daily, but today only once
- Lots of flatulence
- Generalised spasmodic pain in abdomen; worse when eating

Diet

- No gluten, no sugar
- Drinking milk; not having any problems

Explanation

Diet

There are still bowel symptoms present, and the consumption of milk could be an aggravating factor. The patient seems to think it is not affecting her in spite of the symptoms of spasm, flatulence and frequent bowel movements.

Thyroid

The GP was confused as to why the patients TSH had risen, but she was losing weight and not gaining weight. Serum TSH does not give an accurate representation of what is happening with the thyroid peripherally. The issues with serum levels of hormones have been discussed in previous chapters. Functional biology is needed in order to correctly evaluate the cellular activity of the hormones, and to assess the role played by the other endocrine axes in the disorder at hand. Unfortunately, the patient was not able to have a functional biology at that time.

It is important to note that emotional stress is a major aggressor which affects the evolution of Crohn's disease. Something I see very often in my clinic. As mentioned before. Patients with autoimmune disease are very sensitive people. I find that in these patients it is not a simple question of hyperactive immunity, their whole system is overactive, hyperreactive on a physical and emotional level.

Treatment

Repeat all previously prescribed supplements.

Added in

- B-complex and B5 500 mg bid
- Advised patient stick to recommended diet and to eat regular meals
  B5 was added to further support adrenals.

Rx.3

Viburnum opulus	25 ml
Hydrastis canadensis	20 ml
Artemisia absinthium	5 ml

Chamomilla recutita	25 ml
Glycyrrhiza glabra 1:3	15 ml
Melissa officinalis	20 ml
Rehmannia glutinosa prepared root	10 ml

Sig: 8.5 ml bd

Rationale for prescription

Decided to remove *Vitex* and *Lithospermum* as they were part of the formulation for a while and without the functional biology results it is not possible to assess exactly what is occurring at the level of the gonadotropic axis. Removed the *Agrimonia* and increased the dose of *Viburnum* to provide greater antispasmodic action. Added *Melissa* as an alphasympatholytic, GABA-ergic and antispasmodic. *Melissa* is useful for relaxing the sphincter of Oddi, so is useful in cases of splanchnic congestion. *Rehmannia* for adrenal support.

Follow-up appointment 6 weeks later

- Skin in general has been better and has not required moisturiser.
- Finished quercetin and turmeric supplements, has not had any allergic reactions at all. Lips are okay.
- Has had a repeat blood test with the GP and TSH results all normal. Is maintaining 100 micrograms thyroxin.
- The patient feels she is managing stress better than before and is feeling calmer. Weight has stabilised, and no further weight loss, but seems to notice losing some body fat.
- The patient feels flatulence is a problem at the moment.
- Blood pressure: 105/70.

Sleep

- Sleeping well and feels rested

Diet

- Not eating very much, but is having healthy food
- Is now having breakfast, and smaller meals and more often

GIT

- No general cramps, but will get some with eating
- Experiencing a bit of wind; less than before

- No bleeding
- Opens bowels once or twice daily

Treatment

- Repeat all supplements previously taking
- Repeat Rx.3 but replaced *Hydrastis* with *Andrographis*
- The patient has started using a multivitamin

Added in

- Biocare bioenzyme

Sig: 1 bid with food
Digestive Enzyme to support the pancreas and to reduce flatulence.

Follow-up appointment 6 weeks later

- Skin is overall good recently. No swelling or stinging lips. No allergic responses.
- Had a reaction after eating prawns on two occasions. Advised patient to stay off them for now. Has regained about 10 lbs in weight.
- Experienced a little constipation with green clay on one occasion, followed by loose stools, but occurred a day after eating gluten.
- Feeling good about things. Is considering ceasing use of cetirizine.

GIT

- No problems with bowels
- No blood in stools; no mucus
- Opening bowels once daily
- Wind has settled down; only present with certain foods/drinks, e.g. fizzy drinks

Treatment

- Repeat all previous supplements prescribed
- Repeat Rx.3

Summary

I have treated and kept an eye on this patient for many years. She is generally very well and not taking any allopathic medication for Crohn's disease. There have been two instances over the years of intense, stressful periods which have resulted in flare-ups of her Crohn's, but they are short-lived and have settled within a few weeks of herbal treatment. She is generally not on any herbal treatment long term and is enjoying life. I would have liked her to be stricter with her diet, especially in the early part of treatment but as a practitioner, you need to work with what the patient is willing to do and see what results are achievable.

Case 8

A 57-year-old female. Cholecystectomy approximately 8 weeks ago, initial symptoms of pain improved after surgery. One month after surgery, developed lots of pain in the epigastric region; managed with tramadol but resulted in constipation and distension. Having to use laxatives. Symptoms include spasmodic pain which can be recurring, in one instance lasted 5 hours, distention of the abdomen, shaking of arms and legs with the pain and palpitation. Has had seven episodes of this spasmodic pain over the month.

Also presenting with endometriosis; treated with Provera for 8 years, which has been helpful. Diagnosed with IBS; continued diarrhoea. Last year bad case of vestibular hypertension with severe dizziness; treated with physical therapy, which was helpful.

In 2011, a vertigo-type problem came on suddenly; shaky and stressed. Had physio—helpful.

Has seen gastroenterologist. Did not do endoscopy as they felt area too inflamed. Performed Computed Tomography (CT) Scan—results were normal. Antidepressants were prescribed; however, the patient does not want to take them. Energy not great, but better than in the past.

Medications

- Ceased all medications (i.e. Provera, on it for 8 years; and Tramadol)
- Previously took omeprazole, ceased (historical reflux; 10 years ago)
- Currently on probiotics
- Taking FOS (fructooligosaccharide)
- Flaxseed oil and evening primrose oil

Sleep

- Dreams a lot, vivid dreams, has always been like that but more recently

Diet

She is a vegetarian but will eat eggs and fish. Is also restricted to what can east due to spasmodic pain and distention.

- Banana and yofu tofu (soya yoghurt), oat cereals, peppermint tea
- No snacks; doesn't drink coffee
- Lunch: porridge with yofu, anchovies, salad, corn cakes, rice cakes eggs, goat's cheese, brown rice
- Can't tolerate raw fruits; can have stewed apples, apricots and sultanas as anything more effects bowels

Findings

- Eyelids tremble when closed +++
- Lots of skin redness ++++
- Cold and clammy hands and feet +++
- Unable to examine abdomen fully due to surgery being only 8 weeks ago; epigastric region felt hard and was tender

Explaining the case

This case is very complex in nature. As well as the digestive issues present there is also the long history of endometriosis. With the endometriosis, there will likely be adhesions in multiple places within the abdominal cavity and abdominal organs. For the purpose of this book, we will focus on the main presenting complaint, which is the epigastric pain. The epigastric pain developed a short while after the surgery. Upon palpation, the area was very tight. This is related to the aggression induced by the surgical procedure and hence a high alphasympathetic activity. The high alphasympathetic activity coupled with the high parasympathetic activity is causing the spasm.

In addition to this, adhesions may be present. As discussed previously; the research shows that 90% of patients who have abdominal surgery develop adhesions. The surgical procedure, having been performed recently means that these adhesions may be in the early stages of formation and may not be well developed. This is something that a manual therapist, who specialises in this field will have to assess. We can conclude that there exists a spasmodic phenomenon that may be in part related to the early formation of adhesions but is certainly related to imbalances at the level of the autonomic nervous system. Judging by the patient's history, there already existed specific imbalances along the endocrine and autonomic nervous system which predisposed her to such problems. This is what we call the pre-critical terrain.

The palpitations and shaking are caused by the reactive beta discharge (TRH and adrenalin), moments of exaggerated beta response due to the very high alphasympathetic activity. There could be instability in the patient's blood glucose levels due to the endocrine and autonomic nervous system issues, but we need a functional biology test to confirm this. The elevated histamine (autacoid of alpha) exacerbates the problem, as it reinforces alphasympathetic activity. It is a factor that makes the patient more sensitive to pain.

The patient did have a CT scan which did not identify any abnormalities. Computed Tomography is not the best type of scan for looking for adhesions, according to research. In a review of 25 studies, comparing the accuracy of CT, Magnetic Resonance Imaging (MRI) and Ultrasound (US) the results were as such: US—between 76 and 100%. MRI—between 79 and 90% and CT 66%. The study concluded that US and MRI are better at imaging and therefore, diagnosing adhesions. US is useful for imaging adhesions between the bowel and the abdominal wall and MRI for imaging adhesions between the bowel and the abdominal wall but also between the viscera.[230]

Treatment plan

- Reduce para- and alphasympathetic activity
- Decrease TRH activity
- Support adrenals
- Reduce histamine
- Reduce inflammation
- Reduce spasm

Advice

- Cut out all refined sugar
- Increase protein
    - try eggs (duck and/or chicken)
    - try some pea or hemp protein twice daily

This is to assist in the healing process after surgery and to help stabilise blood glucose levels.

Treatment

Continue with evening primrose and flaxseed oil.

Rx. 1

Viridian boswellia
Sig: 1 capsule tid
To reduce inflammation.

Rx. 2

Solgar curcumin
Sig: 1 bid
To reduce inflammation.

Rx.3

Chamomilla recutita EO	0.5 ml
Viburnum opulus	25 ml
Paeonia lactiflora	20 ml
Anemone pulsatilla	5 ml
Centella asiatica	20 ml
Thymus vulgaris	15 ml
Angelica sinensis	15 ml

Sig: 5 ml tid

Rational for prescription

Chamomilla EO as an antispasmodic and to reduce para- and alphasympathetic activity. *Thymus* to reduce parasympathetic activity. *Viburnum*, *Paeonia*, *Angelica* and *Anemone* as antispasmodics. *Centella* to assist in the healing of the tissues due to surgery.

Rx.4

Ribes nigrum	100 ml

Sig: 50 gtt bid

Start with ten drops and increase gradually. Increase by 10 gtt every 5 days until reaching 50 gtt.

To support adrenals. With patients that are sensitive and also present with palpitations, it is important to increase the *Ribes* slowly. If too much is used, it can cause more palpitation as it reinforces beta activity.

Rx.5

Try Better You magnesium spray on abdomen and legs, etc.

Magnesium is highly beneficial when there is spasm present. I have found it to be indispensable with patients who have spasmophilia.

Follow-up appointment 2.5 weeks later

Generally feeling a lot better; has been able to do some work. Has started taking *Viridian quercetin* B5 complex 2 capsules bid as recommended on the telephone as had very itchy skin. Feels it helped immediately. Not taking laxatives now. At first, constipation got worse, but then improved. Seems to be getting a reaction to the magnesium spray. Can irritate the skin in certain places. Energy and stamina much better and concentration has improved. Feels herbal medicine has helped a lot with shaking.

Upon examination, the epigastric region felt softer than it was initially. No nausea or vomiting. Palpitations reduced. About 3–4 times in the last 2 weeks felt 'heart pounding' and could hear it in her ear. Blood pressure: 105/68.

Blood test results of liver function from before and after surgery showed raised enzymes:

- Gamma GT 153; range 6–42
- Aspartate transaminase 33; range 0–31
- Alanine aminotransferase 67; range 10–35

GIT

- Some swelling of the abdomen in evenings, but better than before. Swelling improves by the morning.
- Flatulence is better.

Diet

- Having a fig and prunes at night and linseed in the mornings; helping to regulate bowels.
- Eating more protein; eating tofu and eggs but can't have eggs too often as can be constipating. Has goat's cheese, increased brazil nuts and almonds.
- Taking pea protein three times per week.

Treatment

Repeat

- Magnesium oil spray
- *Boswellia* sig: 1 qid
- *Curcumin*
- Quercetin B5 Complex
- Rx.4

Prescribed Lamberts ibizine
Sig: 1 bid
This is a high potency artichoke extract to support liver function.

Rx.3

Chamomilla recutita EO	0.5 ml
Viburnum opulus	20 ml

Paeonia lactiflora	15 ml
Anemone pulsatilla	5 ml
Centella asiatica	20 ml
Thymus vulgaris	15 ml
Angelica sinensis	15 ml
Glycyrrhiza glabra 1:3	15 ml

Sig: 5 ml tid

Rationale for prescription

Changed quantities of the plants used to make space for *Glycyrrhiza* in order to support adrenals more.

Follow-up appointment 3 weeks later

Opening bowels every day; can't remember when last had such good bowel function. Having some hot flushes at night and cold feet in the day. 'Shaky' feeling much better now; not shaking at all. This shaky feeling was present before the surgery as well patient said. Not just related to epigastric pain.

Started taking probiotic; 20 billion in one capsule, once or twice daily. The only issue remaining now is abdominal distention. Not daily, only happening sometimes.

Findings

- Less tenderness and softer feeling generally over the abdomen.
- Tenderness in the solar plexus region and in the umbilical region due to scar from laparoscopy.
- Eyelids tremble when closed +++. Reports lots of vivid dreams, always been like that.
- Very cold feet and hands +++.
- Dampness of hands ++, an improvement from the last examination.
- Tongue, a little white coating.

Piles

- Using cortisone cream
- Bleeding improved

Advised

- Check liver function in 2 months
- Stay off refined sugar
- Suggest myofascial release to assist in treating adhesion

The patient is taking evening primrose oil 500 mg six times daily.

Treatment

Repeat

- Magnesium oil spray
- *Boswellia* sig: 1 qid
- *Curcumin*
- Quercitin B5 complex
- Ibizine
- Probiotic
- Rx.4

Rx.3

Lavandula angustifolia EO	1 ml
Viburnum opulus	20 ml
Paeonia lactiflora	15 ml
Vitex agnus-castus	7 ml
Anemone pulsatilla	5 ml
Centella asiatica	20 ml
Thymus vulgaris	15 ml
Angelica sinensis	15 ml
Glycyrrhiza glabra 1:1	15 ml
Fabiana imbricata	10 ml

Sig: 8 ml bid

Rationale for prescription

Removed *Chamomilla* EO and used *Lavandula* EO as it is a stronger alphasympatholytic plant. Added *Fabiana* to reduce TRH activity.

Rx.8

Massage oil

Hypericum perforatum macerated oil	60 ml
Chamomilla recutita EO	1 ml
Levisticum officinale EO	1 ml
Lavandula angustifolia EO	2 ml
Thymus vulgaris ct linalool EO	1 ml
Angelica archangelica tincture	5 ml

Sig: massage the epigastric area for 10 minutes bid in a downward and outward motion following the line of the rib cage, but not over the rib cage, just below the rib cage

Rationale for prescription

The essential oils in this preparation are capable of penetrating the skin and being absorbed into the body will have a local and systemic effect, if used long term. The aim here was to use EO's that have para- and alphasympatholytic properties to help prevent spasm and relax the tissues. *Chamomilla*: antispasmodic, para- and alphasympatholytic. *Lavandula*: strong alphasympatholytic, *Thymus*: strongly parasympatholytic, *Levisticum*: para- and alphasympatholytic. Angelica: antispasmodic.

Follow-up appointment 1 month later

Bowels are very regular now. The shaking has gone completely. Has been able to do much more work, plus walking and exercise. Has good energy levels. Feels massage with lotion has really helped to free up the epigastric region. Feels abdominal issues are so much better and no longer problematic. The main problem now is managing endometriosis. Liver function was retested after 2 months of treatment, and all the enzymes were normal.

Case 9

A 14-year-old male presenting with Crohn's disease, which was diagnosed 2 years ago. Colonoscopy performed at the time revealed ulceration. The patient is unaware of the location of Crohn's relative to the bowel.

Chronic blood loss resulted in anaemia and had to have a transfusion approx. 6 months ago. Symptoms include opening bowels 5–6 times daily; watery stools with undigested food and blood. Abdominal pain present with or without passing stools but not consistently.

History: born by C-section, breastfed for 8 months. Mother says he did not have any problems as a baby. All vaccines given as a child. Previously on azathioprine for 1 week but reacted badly: fever and raised liver enzymes. The consultant wanted to try him on mercaptopurine instead. Patient and parents did not want to try any more allopathic medication.

Medications

- Asacol (mesalazine) tabs: 400 mg 2 tid
- Sytron sodium feredetate: 5 ml bid
- Lamberts Acidophilus extra 10: 1 od

Diet

Very fussy eater. Does not eat vegetables as does not like them.

- Breakfast: cheese on toast
- Lunch: baguette at school

- Snacks: gluten-free crackers, bananas
- Dinner: chicken, rice, gluten-free pasta, chips

Findings

- Some ulcerations in the mouth, does not look like Crohn's disease
- Adrenal congestion +++
- Splanchnic congestion +++
- Cold hands and feet +++
- Damp hands and feet ++
- Tongue white +++
- Abdomen tenders in the ileocecal region and descending colon

Explaining the case

It is important to look at the complete history of the patient in order to understand the factors that may have led to the development of the disease. This patient was born by caesarean, which is an important factor in the initial development of the microbiome. The bacteria from the birthing canal were not provided. It would have been beneficial to have had more information on the childhood period, but this information was not provided. Sometimes parts of the history are forgotten, and the information is not available.

The patient's age is significant. He is 14 years old but was diagnosed 2 years ago, so was approximately 12 years old when the symptoms started. This is the age when puberty begins, and as a result profound changes occur at the level of the endocrine and autonomic nervous systems. The organism is establishing a new way of functioning. This brings into play the syndrome of adaptation. The adrenals are under more strain to help the organism adapt to this new way of functioning. All of the other endocrine axes will be affected to some degree due to puberty and growth. This is why a functional biology is necessary in order to establish the factors at play.

The patient's diet is not good. It is high in carbohydrates which trigger insulin and thus participate in inflammation. In addition to this, they can disrupt the microbiome, promoting pathogenic bacteria and thus inflammation by other means.

Treatment plan

- Reduce alpha and parasympathetic activity
- Decongest splanchnic region; drain the pancreas
- Support adrenals

- Restore balance to the microbiome
- Reduce inflammation and heal gastrointestinal mucosa

Treatment

Advised GAPS diet. Start with stage one and assess symptoms in a week or two. Advised patient when possible to have a functional biology blood test.

Rx.1

Green clay
Sig: 1 tsp od or bd
Used as an anti-inflammatory for the GI system.

Rx.2

Hydrastis canadensis	20 ml
Ribes nigrum	30 ml
Glycyrrhiza glabra 1:3	20 ml
Chamomilla recutita	30 ml
Sig: 7.5 ml bid	

Rationale for prescription

Used *Hydrastis* as a mucous membrane restorative, anti-inflammatory and astringent. *Ribes* to support adrenal glands. *Glycyrrhiza* to support adrenal glands and as an anti-inflammatory. *Chamomilla* to reduce para and alphasympathetic activity and as an anti-inflammatory. Pancreatic drainage will be addressed later on in the treatment.

Rx.3

Viridian boswellia capsules
Sig: 1 bid, slowly increase to 3 bid
As an anti-inflammatory.

Rx.4

Probiotics: either prescript biotic or megaspore biotic
To correct the imbalance in the microbiome.

Follow-up appointment 1 month later

- Following stage 1 of the GAPS diet, he is drinking meat stock regularly. Eating chicken and meat, broccoli heads, carrots, green beans for approximately 3 weeks now.

- Taking the supplements but not the herbal tincture (No.2). Does not like the taste.
- Sometimes feels tired, low energy. Seems to be hungry all the time.
- Has reduced the amount of exercise; not doing PE or playing football now.

GIT

- Opening bowels up to three times daily; reduced from up to six times
- No blood in stools now
- No pain in bowels now when passing stools

Findings

- No ulcerations in mouth. Cleared up
- Tongue still white +++

Diet, add in on a 3-day cycle to test if tolerated:

- Egg yolks, then whites
- Pumpkin and butternut squash
- Avocado
- Kale
- Onion
- Coconut oil

Treatment

Carry on with all prescriptions and discussed the importance of taking the herbal tincture.

Follow-up appointment 1 month later

- Seeing improvements; opening bowels 1–2 times daily. Little cramping when opens bowels. The pain stops once finished opening bowels. Had a bit of popcorn once and then had some bleeding; stopped the next day.
- Energy has improved. Not as hungry as used to be.
- Has been managing to take 7.5ml bid of herbal medicine now.

Diet

- On stage 3 of GAPS diet
- Having homemade yoghurt; avocado, chicken, eggs, beef, lamb, squash, spinach. Not eating many other vegetables as does not like vegetables

Advised that it is important to increase the variety of vegetables consumed.

- Consider roasted pumpkin
- Try baked apple and stewed pear
- In 2–3 weeks try to move onto stage 4 of GAPS diet

Treatment

Repeat all medications as previously.

Rx.2

Hydrastis canadensis	20 ml
Plantago major	20 ml
Agrimonia eupatoria	10 ml
Chamomilla recutita	30 ml
Glycyrrhiza glabra 1:1	20 ml
Sig: 7.5 ml bid	

Rationale for prescription

Switched to *Glycyrrhiza* 1:1 as is stronger. Added *Agrimonia* to drain pancreas and indirectly reduces parasympathetic activity by supporting pancreas. Added *Plantago* for its intestinal drainage properties; astringent. Plantago is also a pancreatic drainer.

Rx. 5

Ribes nigrum	100 ml
Sig: slowly increase to 100 gtt bid	

Removed from Rx.2 to make space for other herbs. *Ribes* was used to support adrenals.

Follow-up appointment 5 weeks later

- Feeling well. Energy is good; has gone back to playing football now.
- Opening bowels once a day and no blood. On a 'bad' day opens bowels twice a day.
- Little cramping.
- On average has a 'bad' day once a fortnight. Stools are formed now.
- Taking all herbal medicine regularly, including the herbal tincture.
- Grandmother passed away recently, and this was very upsetting for him.
- No appointment with consultants yet. Stopped asacol and iron a while ago. Not on any allopathic medication.

Diet

- On stage 4 of the GAPS diet.
- Eating kale and broccoli heads, spinach, avocado, eggs, homemade yoghurt and is carrying on with the meat stock, etc.

Advised to try

- Garlic and liquid aminos in stir fry
- Cucumber without skin
- Baked apple and stewed pear
- Cooked cabbage
- Celeriac and fennel
- Pure coconut milk

Treatment

Repeat all medications as previously.

Appointment 5 weeks later

Telephoned and said developed an anal abscess. Advised the following prescriptions.

Rx. 1

Colloidal silver spray
Sig: spray on abscess several times daily
Used as an antiseptic agent.

Rx.2

Echinacea premium (mix of *purpurea* and *angustifolia*)	50 ml
Hydrastis canadensis	20 ml
Phytolacca decandra	5 ml
Olea europaea	20 ml
Juglan regia	10 ml
Sig: 5 ml tid	

Rationale for prescription

This formula contains a range of antiseptic and lymphatic plants which were used to help clear the anal abscess. Advised to use this formula for now and stop the other Rx.2 formula.

Rx.3

Lavender EO
Sig: 1–2 drops tid on the abscess
As an anti-inflammatory and antiseptic.

Rx.4

Use green clay as a poultice on the abscess at night. Apply before bed and wash off in the morning.

Clay is a fantastic poultice. It works very quickly, having anti-inflammatory and antibacterial (not all green clays are antibacterial) properties. It draws the toxins out and locks them into its matrix. It is mixed with water or aloe vera juice to form a thick paste. It is then applied fairly thickly to the affected area. It must not dry out, so a damp gauze is placed on top and then a waterproof plaster. If the affected area is on a leg or arm the site can be wrapped.

Continue with all previous supplements and medications apart from old Rx.2 formula as replaced with the above.

Follow-up appointment 3 weeks later

- Abscess almost gone. Has been using all medication prescribed.
- Energy is still good; playing football and not needing to go to the toilet during the game, can go out and do normal activities.

GIT

- Generally, opens bowels once or twice a daily; can get a bit constipated if has too much clay.
- No blood or mucus.
- No cramping now.
- Feels gut is generally good.

Diet

- Following GAPS diet and feels is going well
- Added in stewed pear, coconut milk and using coconut flour
- Advised to try almond butter

Treatment

- Repeat all supplements has been taking but decrease clay to ½ tsp bid
- Repeat Rx.5
- The finish of antiseptic formula Rx.2, then resume old Rx.2

Added in

Lamberts L-glutamine powder
Sig: increase slowly to 1 tsp bid

To assist in repair of the intestinal mucosa.

Follow-up appointment 6 weeks later

Has had stress at school and has been off school for 2 weeks: a boy threatened to fight him. Due to this stress has had some blood in stools, a small amount today and also 1 week ago. Stools got a bit runny, then hard. Opening bowels 1–2 times a day with no mucus. The abscess has completely gone and no pain now.

Diet

- Same as before.
- Advised to add in baked apple as has not tried it yet.
- Has been having Easy-yo yoghurt; contains some sugar and cow's milk. Advised to stop using this and in 3 weeks to try goat's milk kefir.
- Can try banana bread recipe from GAPS book.

Treatment

Repeat all supplements as before

Rx.2

Agrimonia eupatoria	10 ml
Glycyrrhiza glabra 1:1	20 ml
Gentiana lutea	10 ml
Chamomilla recutita	30 ml
Passiflora incarnata	20 ml
Juglans regia	10 ml

Sig: 7.5 ml BD

Rationale for prescription

Increased amount of *Agrimonia*, break from *Hydrastis* as has been taking it for a while, added *Juglans* as a pancreatic drainer, *Passiflora* to further reduce alphasympathetic activity as there has been stress at school. *Gentiana* to reduce parasympathetic activity and also as an effective bitter to support digestion.

Rx.5

Cinnamomum zeylanicum bark EO	1 ml
Lavandula angustifolia EO	1 ml
Ribes nigrum	100 ml

Sig: slowly increase to 100 gtt bid

Added essential oils of *Cinnamomum* and *Lavandula*. *Cinnamomum* to support adrenal glands (only in essential oil form). *Lavandula* as a powerful alphasympatholytic plant.

Follow-up appointment 2 months later

Stopped Easy-yo yoghurt after the last consultation. Bowel movements reduced from 1–2 times daily to every other day. Stools formed sometimes and occasionally a bit runny. No mucus or blood. No stomach pains. Feels well. He has an appointment in March with a consultant.

Energy is very good. Keeping up sports. Played a whole 80 minutes of a football game and seems to be playing faster and harder than ever before; even before being diagnosed with Crohn's, would sometimes 'run out of steam'. Playing a lot of video games, possibly making him stressed.

Findings

- Feet and hands cold +++
- Feet colder than hands
- Hands and feet little damp +
- Adrenal congestion +++
- Splanchnic congestion +++
- Abdomen tender, but better than on the last examination

Treatment

- Advised to try cashew nut butter, lettuce, almonds without skin, walnuts without skin, cauliflower, courgette, asparagus. Try adding cod and haddock to diet.
- Repeat all supplements and herbal tinctures.
- Advised to switch from plain glutamine to planet paleo digestive collagen as it does not only contain glutamine but also other nutrients as well as collagen which are useful for aiding repair of the gastrointestinal mucous membrane.
- Added vitamin D 2000 IU daily and zinc citrate 30 mg; Sig: 1 od noct.

Follow-up appointment 2 months later

- Had another very stressful situation at school, feels this has caused a flare-up of Crohn's. Has been stressed for the last 2 weeks.

- Another abscess has developed—took previous protocol that was prescribed last time had abscess.
- Having an MRI scan in 1 week.
- Returned to stage 1 of GAPS diet due to the return of red blood that carried on. Also was opening bowels up to five times a day. Having cramps and feeling nauseous.

Was offered steroids by his doctor but did not want them. Given Modulen feed to rest the bowel. Has been on this for 1 week. Suggested next time ask for Elemental nutritional therapy instead of Modulen as the ingredients are better. Bleeding generally worse at night but on the whole has reduced.

Treatment

- Repeat all previous supplements.
- Repeat Rx.5.
- Advised to practice abdominal breathing techniques 10 minutes bid to help regulate the autonomic nervous system.
- The patient said will have functional biology test soon.

Rx.2

Hydrastis canadensis	20 ml
Lithospermum officinale	10 ml
Melissa officinalis	20 ml
Agrimonia eupatoria	20 ml
Glycyrrhiza glabra 1:1	20 ml
Viburnum opulus	15 ml
Passiflora incarnata	20 ml
Sig: 6 ml tid	

Rationale for prescription

Changed treatment in light of recent flare-up of Crohn's. Removed *Gentiana*, *Juglans* and *Chamomila*. Increased amount of *Agrimonia*. Added *Viburnum* again as an antispasmodic, *Hydrastis* as an anti-inflammatory, astringent and mucous membrane restorative, *Melissa* as alphasympatholytic and antispasmodic. *Lithospermum* added to reduce FSH which is implicated in autoimmunity.

Follow-up appointment 3 weeks later

Birthday recently, now 15 years old.

Has been using Modulen. Blood had been reducing, but consultant felt that it was not effective enough and convinced him to take prednisolone, eight times 5 mg tablets daily for 1 week (i.e. 40 mg daily) with instructions to reduce slowly before stopping completely. Blood stopped 1 day after starting steroids. Feeling okay taking them. Has been on them for 4 days now. A tiny bit of red blood visible on toilet tissue yesterday, but no other symptoms.

Will see the consultant again in a week. The nurse informed the patient that a recent MRI of his intestines showed some evidence of ulceration. Also, said he has an anal fissure.

Diet

- Back on stage 1 of GAPS diet
- Taking food into school from home

Advised patient to take a thermos into school in order to keep meat stock warm.

Functional biology results: Note that this test was performed before the patient started prednisolone, so it is an accurate representation of what was occurring before the steroids were prescribed.

These are not all of the functional biology indexes. I have selected the most relevant ones related to this case. There are over 150 indexes. As discussed in Chapter 15 there is a Structure (S) value and a Function (F) value. The normal range for each index is listed in the last column.

Table 28. Shows the first set of results of the functional biology

Index	Initial results	Normal range
Cortisol	S 567.8 F 232.4	3–7
Adrenal gland activity	S 319.1 F 53.48	2.7–3.3
Permissivity	S 0.56 F 0.23	0.45–0.8
Adaptation-permissivity	S 248.1 F 178.7	1–3
Histamine activity	S 0.09 F 0.56	36–76
Peripheral serotonin	S 54.53 F 22.32	1.5–7.5
Cata-ana ratio	S 35.22 F 14.42	1.8–3
Inflammation	S 0.04 F 0.11	0.3–2.5

(*Continued*)

Table 28. (Continued)

Index	Initial results	Normal range
Genital ratio	S 0.27 F 0.27	0.8–0.95
Genital estrogens	S 0.05 F 0.18	0.12–0.16
Genital androgens	S 0.02 F 0.07	0.12–0.17
Thyroid metabolic	S 5.82 F 5.82	3.5–5.5
Insulin	S 14.99 F 6.13	1.5–5
Insulin resistance	S 0.01 F 0.03	0.75–1.25

Explaining the functional biology results

When looking at the functional biology results, I always like to remind people that we are not looking at serum levels. We are looking at the activity of the given hormone at a tissular and cellular level. Also, we are looking at the relative activity between one hormone and another.

Corticotropic axis: In this case, we can see that the cortisol index is extremely high, indicating the activity of maladaptive cortisol. The permissivity index is normal in structure and low in function. What is important to note, is that there is a huge cortisol index relative to the permissivity index, which shows that the ratio is in favour of maladaptive cortisol. This is depicted by the elevated adaptation-permissivity index. This has negative metabolic consequences, as we shall discuss now. The expression of histamine is suppressed as the cortisol is so high. Cortisol has a blocking effect on histamine. The high peripheral serotonin index means that central serotonin is low. This affects the emotional state of the patient. The cata/ana ratio index is elevated, and so the patient is more catabolic. The reason for this catabolic activity, which occurs in Crohn's disease, is that there is high cortisol (catabolic hormone). The inflammation index appears low. It is not that there is no inflammation, it is because there is so much cortisol, that it is blocking the expression of inflammation. The inflammatory index appears low as we are looking at it in relative terms. Relative to cortisol. There is in fact inflammatory activity.

Gonadotropic axis: Another reason for the catabolic activity is the low androgens relative to oestrogens, and this is shown by the genital ratio index. Androgens are needed to complete anabolism thus, when they are low relative to oestrogens there is more catabolic activity. You can see that the genital oestrogens are low in structure and this may be confusing in light of what we have just said, but remember it is the relativity which is important. Oestrogens may be low in structure, but if you look at the genital androgens, they are much lower than the oestrogens.

Thyrotropic axis: The thyroid metabolic index is elevated. This implicates the thyroid in the inflammatory process.

Somatotropic axis: Here we can see that the insulin index is elevated and the insulin resistance index is low, showing that insulin is very high. We have discussed the role that insulin plays in inflammation (increasing it) and increasing free radical activity.

This patient is worse in structure and better in function. This means that the patient is better when engaging in the world rather than going inside himself. With patients like this, I do not recommend that they meditate for long, as when they meditate, they go inside themselves and their biochemistry changes for the worse. Activity is better for them, so I encourage them to practice something like Tai Chi or moving Qigong exercises. It is important for them to be mindful of their breath and their movements in order to rebalance the organism. A person can perform a movement, but if they are thinking of their problems or what they need to do later on while training, then they will not relax. They are not really changing their state. As these patients are better in function, the movement helps them focus their mind on something and not their problems, but they still need to train their focus and keep bringing their mind back to the movement and the breath. For patients that are more balanced between structure and function or are better in structure, then a sitting, closed-eyed meditation is okay for them. I find that in patients that are still growing, it is easier to balance the ratio of structure and function. In older patients, it is much harder and takes longer to change.

Treatment plan

- Reduce maladaptive cortisol and reduce the ratio of maladaptive to permissive cortisol
- Support the adrenals as they are so overworked
- Reduce para- and alphasympathetic activity
- Increase central serotonin
- Drain pancreas
- Reduce thyroid activity as it participates in inflammation
- Increase genital androgens
- Reduce inflammation
- Reduce insulin activity
- Reduce FSH activity
- Reduce spasm
- Provide healing for gut mucosa
- Restore microbiome

Treatment

Repeat

- Green clay
- *Viridian boswellia* capsules
- Take probiotic; megaspore biotic

Rx. 1

Chamomilla recutita EO	1 ml
Lavandula angustifolia EO	1 ml
Agrimonia eupatoria	20 ml
Ribes nigrum	30 ml
Vitex agnus-castus	10 ml
Withania somnifera	25 ml
Melissa officinalis	20 ml
Artemisia absinthium	5 ml
Lycopus europaeus	10 ml

Sig: 8.5 ml tid

Rationale for prescription

Chamomilla EO used to reduce para- and alphasympathetic activity. *Lavandula* as a potent alphasympatholytic. *Agrimonia* to drain the pancreas, as an anti-inflammatory and indirectly reduces parasympathetic activity by supporting the pancreas. *Ribes* to support adrenals. *Vitex* to reduce FSH activity. FSH plays a major role in autoimmunity, as discussed previously. *Withania* to improve genital androgens, also as an adaptogen it will help regulate cortisol. *Melissa* as an alphasympatholytic and antispasmodic. *Lycopus* to reduce thyroid activity. Artemisia for its benefits in treating Crohn's disease, as discussed previously.

Rx.2

Biocare 5-HTP 50 mg
Sig: 1 bid away from food, morning and evening
To increase central serotonin.

Rx.3

Herbal Infusion
Plantago major

Chamomilla recutita
Passiflora incarnata
Sig: 1 tsp aa tid as infusion

Plantago as intestinal drainer, pancreatic drainer, anti-inflammatory. *Chamomilla* to reduce para- and alphasympathetic activity, anti-inflammatory and antispasmodic. *Passiflora* as an alphasympatholytic.

Rx.5

Malva sylvestris   100 ml
Sig: 30 gtt tid to be taken after each meal

Malva is used for reducing insulin. It is better to use it after a meal due to insulin stimulation when eating. In some patients that are not compliant I sometimes mix it into the formulation that is taken before food.

Rx.7

Curcumin x 4000
Sig: 2 bid
As an anti-inflammatory.

Rx.8

Biocare mega EPA—fish oil supplement
Sig: 1 bid
As an anti-inflammatory.

Rx.9

Tigon eden extract
Sig: start with 1 bid and increase slowly to 2 tid

This is a very potent olive leaf supplement which I find very useful in dealing with conditions where there is dysbiosis and inflammation of the bowel. It is a potent anti-fungal, antibacterial and antiviral. Olive leaves are an effective anti-inflammatory and antioxidant.

Follow-up appointment 3 months later

• Came off steroids 3 weeks ago.
• Has put on weight. Now 9.10 stone. Energy has returned.

- No stress at the moment.
- Parents say, can be a problem getting him to stop playing computer games; can play them all day.

Diet

- Grilled lamb, chicken, fish, meatballs
- Butternut squash, cucumber, broccoli heads
- Ripe bananas, coconut milk, avocados

Advised to try green beans, activated nuts (almonds, walnuts, pecans), lettuce and mushroom.

GIT

- Opens bowels once daily, only in the morning. Stools often formed.
- No gas.
- No blood or mucous for 3 months, with the exception of 3 weeks ago a speck of blood on tissue from anal fissure.
- Stools can sometimes be hard.

Was examined by a specialist; abscess has healed but could see the anal fissure.

Advice

Reduce computer games as they are a source of stress. They increase alphasympathetic activity.

Treatment

- Carry on with fish oil for 3 months then stop
- Finish off the supply of Eden extract then stop
- Repeat all other medication

Follow-up appointment 3 months later

Right knee suddenly became swollen 1 week ago, and parents feel there was no obvious reason for it. Some puss was coming out from a very small spot on the knee.

Parents say there is no major stress. GP prescribed antibiotics, but he has not used them yet. Wants to avoid taking them. Is able to walk. Knee not currently painful but was before. Has used green clay poultice and frankincense essential oil for three nights as advised by me on the telephone and swelling has been coming down.

GIT

- Opening bowels once or twice daily
- No mucous, little red blood but feels is likely from fissure

Advised to try using 1 gtt of *Lavandula* EO neat on the area where anal fissure is.

The reason why anal fissures are hard to heal is that the sphincter is always under a level of constriction and this affects the flow of blood to the area, thus affecting healing. If you are able to relax the sphincter to some degree and improve blood flow to the area they usually heal well.

Diet

- GAPS diet as previously

Advised to add in

- Coconut milk curry
- Fatty meats, e.g. pork belly, lamb shank etc.
- Hemp oil, avocado oil, olive and coconut oil
- Deseeded tomatoes
- Smooth peanut butter
- Stewed apples

Treatment

- Repeat all supplements and herbal medicines, but changed Rx.1 as below.
- Break from *Curcumin* × 4000 and switch back to *Boswellia* capsules.

Advised to use

- Serraenzyme: Sig: 1 bid 1 hour before food and slowly increase to 2–3 bid
- Carry on with green clay poultice at night

Serraenzyme is a valuable anti-inflammatory enzyme useful for many inflammatory conditions. I prescribed this to help with the swelling in the knee. It must be taken away from food.

Rx.1

Chamomilla recutita EO	1 ml
Lavandula angustifolia EO	1 ml

Quercus spiritus glandium D3	10 ml
Echinacea premium	20 ml
Lycopus europaeus	10 ml
Withania somnifera	25 ml
Ribes nigrum	30 ml
Glycyrrhiza glabra 1:3	10 ml
Hydrastis canadensis	20 ml

Sig: 8.5 ml td

Rationale for prescription

Echinacea was used for the infection in the knee and as a lymphatic cleanser. *Hydrastis* as anti-inflammatory and antibacterial. *Glycyrrhiza* as an anti-inflammatory and to support adrenals. Quercus to reduce peripheral oestrogen activity.

Follow-up appointment 1 month later

- Swelling in right knee improved within 1 week, then left knee got swollen and hamstring tightness. Had a few days off school. Swelling then came down. No pain in knees now and barely swollen.
- Has had stress due to mock exams coming up.
- Fissure not painful but did see some red blood sometimes.

GIT

- Had some cheese and sweets on Halloween and since then, the bowel has been irritated. Softer, sometimes watery stools
- One day opened bowels four times, other days 2–3 times
- Is just now calming down and regulating

Diet

- Has added in smooth peanut butter, coconut milk, fatty meat, pork belly etc. and is all okay
- Didn't try hemp oil or deseeded tomato yet
- Having greens and green leafy veg

Advised to add in

- Red and green peppers and spring onion and see if tolerated

Functional biology results

Table 29. Shows the results of the functional biology after approx. 6 months of treatment

Index	Initial results	Results after 6 months of treatment	Normal range
Cortisol	S 567.8 F 232.4	S 84 F 79.34	3–7
Adrenal gland activity	S 319.1 F 53.48	S 27.28 F 24.34	2.7–3.3
Permissivity	S 0.56 F 0.23	S 0.32 F 0.31	0.45–0.8
Adaptation-permissivity	S 248.1 F 178.7	S 56.39 F 54.69	1–3
Histamine activity	S 0.09 F 0.56	S 1.45 F 1.63	36–76
Peripheral serotonin	S 54.53 F 22.32	S 20.72 F 19.57	1.5–7.5
Cata-ana ratio	S 35.22 F 14.42	S 11.09 F 10.48	1.8–3
Inflammation	S 0.04 F 0.11	S 0.04 F 0.04	0.3–2.5
Genital ratio	S 0.27 F 0.27	S 0.43 F 0.43	0.8–0.95
Genital estrogens	S 0.05 F 0.18	S 0.17 F 0.18	0.12–0.16
Genital androgens	S 0.02 F 0.07	S 0.10 F 0.10	0.12–0.17
Thyroid metabolic	S 5.82 F 5.82	S 2.31 F 2.31	3.5–5.5
Insulin	S 14.99 F 6.13	S 1.90 F 1.79	1.5–5
Insulin resistance	S 0.01 F 0.03	S 0.24 F 0.27	0.75–1.25

Explaining the functional biology results

Corticotropic axis: After 6 months of treatment, there has been a considerable reduc-tion in the cortisol index, along with a reduction in the adrenal gland activity index. The adaptation-permissivity index has reduced from 248.1 to 56.39 in structure, sig-nifying that there is now much less maladaptive to permissive cortisol. There is more balance. The permissivity index has dropped a little in structure, but has risen in function. What is more important, though, and as mentioned, is that the ratio of maladaptive to permissive cortisol has improved. The histamine activity has increased as the cortisol has reduced, so again, you can see the connection between the two. Peripheral serotonin has reduced, which means that central serotonin has increased.

The inflammation index is stable in structure and has reduced slightly in function. The inflammatory activity which occurs in the organism is a complex process, and many hormones are implicated in the process, for example, insulin. Therefore, it is necessary to evaluate multiple indexes in the functional biology and their effect upon one another.

As the cortisol has decreased, the cata/ana ratio has as well. There is now less catabolic activity than previously.

Gonadotropic axis: There is also less catabolic activity as genital androgens have risen relative to oestrogens. This is evident by the rise in the genital ratio index.

Thyrotropic axis: The thyroid metabolic activity has decreased but is now lower than the normal range. The treatment needs to be adjusted.

Somatotropic axis: The insulin index has now normalised, and the insulin resistance index has increased. This is positive, as there will be less inflammatory activity.

Overall the difference between structure and function has changed considerably. This implies, that the organism is much more balanced and stable than previously.

Treatment

- Carry on with all previous supplements and herbal preparations
- Take vitamin D 2000 IU daily
- Switch *Boswellia* capsules to Mediherb *Boswellia* complex tablets; Sig: 1 tid

Boswellia complex tablets contain therapeutic doses of *Curcuma*, *Boswellia*, *Zingiber* and *Apium*. It is an effective anti-inflammatory as all the ingredients work synergistically.

Rx. 1

Chamomilla recutita EO	1 ml
Lavandula angustifolia EO	1 ml
Eschscholzia californica	20 ml
Withania somnifera	25 ml
Ribes nigrum	30 ml
Glycyrrhiza glabra 1:3	15 ml
Vitex agnus-castus	10 ml
Fucus vesiculosus	20 ml
Artemisia absinthium	5 ml

Sig: 8.5 ml bid

Rationale for prescription

Removed *Lycopus* and *Melissa* as the thyroid metabolic activity has dropped. Added *Fucus* to improve peripheral thyroid activity. *Eschscholzia* used for its sympatholytic effect.

Follow-up appointment 2 months later

- Developed rash all over hands following consumption of garlic sauce from a take-away meal. GP prescribed antihistamines but has not taken them.
- Advised to take Solgar quercetin complex 1 tid and following formula to reduce histamine.

Formula to reduce histamine

Albizia lebbeck	25 ml
Plantago major	25 ml
Sig: 60 gtt tid	

Follow-up appointment 2.5 weeks later

- Took 3–4 days for the rash to settle with herbal medication. Swelling in knees has gone completely now.
- Energy is good. Has noticed that if he has a nap in the afternoon, upon waking will need to open bowels. Now naps twice a week, on Wing Chun training days.
- Going to bed late. 12.30 for no known reason. Is simply playing on the phone. Seems to be a deep sleeper.
- Started MMA (Mixed Martial Arts) training but will probably stop this as it interferes with Wing Chun training plus is receiving some blows to the abdomen and this is not good for him.
- Possibly a bit stressed. Recently not able to control anger well and has gotten very angry easily. Is studying for GCSE's this year and does not want to do them.
- Weight is good. Has gone up a bit.

GIT

- Normally opens bowels once a day and stools are formed nine out of ten times
- On occasions, stools can be a bit loose

Diet

- Added in peppers and is okay with them
- Has not yet tried deseeded tomato, hemp oil or spring onion

Treatment

- Advised to stop serraenzyme now
- Advised if wanting to use fish oil to take it on and off, not continuously
- Repeat all previous supplements and herbal medicines apart from serraenzyme
- Advised to take Zinc citrate 30 mg. Sig: 1 od

I generally don't give fish oils for more than 6 months without checking essential fatty acid status.

I am still treating this patient. He is making steady progress, as seen from his functional biology results and case notes. It takes time to treat the underlying endocrine and autonomic nervous system imbalances, but if the treatment is correct and if the patient is willing to do what is needed, it is quite fascinating as to what can be achieved.

REFERENCE LIST

1. Gibson, M. K., Crofts, T. S., & Dantas, G. (2015). Antibiotics and the developing infant gut microbiota and resistome. *Curr Opin Microbiol*, 27: 51–56. doi: 10.1016/j.mib.2015.07.007. E-pub: 1 August 2015.
2. Marlicz, W. (2014). Nonsteroidal anti-inflammatory drugs, proton pump inhibitors, and gastrointestinal injury: Contrasting interactions in the stomach and small intestine. *Mayo Clinic Proceedings*, 89(12): 1699–1709.
3. Gross, L., & Birnbaum, L. S. (2018). Regulating toxic chemicals for public and environmental health Published: *PLOS Biology*, 16(1): e100261. https://journals.plos.org/plosbiology/article?id=10.1371/journal.pbio.1002619.
4. Nandipati, S., & Litvan, I. *International Journal of Environmental research and Public Health*. Review Environmental Exposures and Parkinson's Disease. Department of Neurosciences Movement Disorders Center, University of California, San Diego. Academic Editor: Paul B. Tchounwou. Received: 6 May 2016. Accepted: 30 August 2016. Published: 3 September 2016.
5. *American Journal of Pharmaceutical Education*. (2007). 71(4): Article 78.
6. Pakala, R. S., & Brown, K. N. *Cholinergic Medications*. Augusta University. Last update: 20 February 2019. https://www.ncbi.nlm.nih.gov/books/NBK538163/.
7. http://www.pathwaymedicine.org/parasympathetic-nervous-system.
8. Breit, S., Kupferberg, A., Rogler, G., & Hasle, G. (2018). Frontiers in psychiatry. Vagus nerve as modulator of the brain–gut axis in psychiatric and inflammatory disorders. *Front Psychiatry*, 9: 44. Published online: 13 March 2018.
9. Pruessner, J. C., Champagne, F., Meaney, M. J., & Dagher, A. (2004). Behavioral/systems/cognitive dopamine release in response to a psychological stress in humans and its relationship to early life maternal care: A positron emission tomography study using [^{11}C], Raclopride. *Journal of Neuroscience*, 24(11): 2825–2831.

10. Siegel, A., & Victoroff, J. (2009). Understanding human aggression: New insights from neuroscience. *International Journal of Law and Psychiatry, 32*(4): 209–215.

11. Verberne, A. J. M., Korim, W. S., Sabetghadam, A., & Llewellyn-Smith, I. J. (2016). Adrenaline: insights into its metabolic roles in hypoglycaemia and diabetes. *Br J Pharmacol, 173*(9): 1425–1437. Published online: 8 March 2016. doi: 10.1111/bph.13458.

12. Gardner, D., & Shoback, D. (2007). *Greenspan's Basic & Clinical Endocrinology.* Eighth edition. The McGraw-Hill Companies. United States.

13. Notes from Dr Lapraz: seminar on autonomic nervous system.

14. *Journal of autacoids and hormones.* https://www.omicsonline.org/autacoids-and-hormones.php.

15. Coussons-Read, M. E. (2013). Effects of prenatal stress on pregnancy and human development: mechanisms and pathways. The royal society of medicine journals. *Obstet Med, 6*(2): 52–57. Published online: 3 May 2013.

16. Dave, N. D., MBBS, Clinical fellow, Lianbin Xiang, MD, Assistant Professor of Medicine, Kristina E. Rehm, PhD, Postdoctoral Research Fellow, and Gailen D. Marshall, Jr., MD, PhD, Professor of Medicine and Paediatrics. Stress and Allergic Diseases. *Immunol Allergy Clin North Am.* Author manuscript. Available in PMC: 1 February 2012. Published in final edited form as: *Immunol Allergy Clin North Am.* February 2011; *31*(1):55–68.

17. https://www.britannica.com/science/histamine.

18. Ramesh, V. et al. (2004). Wakefulness-inducing effects of histamine in the basal forebrain of freely moving rats. *Behavioural Brain Research, 152*(2): 271–278.

19. Eutamene, H. (2003). Acute stress modulates the histamine content of mast cells in the gastrointestinal tract through interleukin-1 and corticotropin-release in rats. *J Physiol, 553*(Pt 3): 959–966.

20. Petra, C., et al. (2006). Neuroimmunology of stress: Skin takes center stage. *J Invest Dermatol, 126*(8): 1697–1704.

21. Jutel, M., Blaser, K., & Akdis, C. A. (2006). The role of histamine in regulation of immune responses. *Chem Immunol Allergy, 91*: 174–187.

22. Jutel, M., Watanabe, T., Klunker, S., Akdis, M., Thomet, O. A., Malolepszy, J., Zak-Nejmark, T., Koga, R., Kobayashi, T., Blaser, K., & Akdis, C. A. (2001). Histamine regulates T-cell and antibody responses by differential expression of H1 and H2 receptors. *Nature, 413*(6854): 420–425.

23. Haas, H. L., Sergeeva, O. A., & Selbach, O. Histamine in the nervous system. American physiological society. 1 July 2008. doi:10.1152/physrev.00043.2007.

24. Notes from Dr Lapraz: seminar on serotonin and para-sympathetic activity.

25. Duraffourd, C., & Lapraz. J.-C. *Traité de phytothérapie clinique*, Masson, Paris, 2002.

26. Scaglione, F., & Zangara, A. *Journal of Sleep Disorders And Management.* Research Article. Valeriana Officinalis and Melissa Officinalis Extracts Normalize Brain Levels of GABA and Glutamate Altered by Chronic Stress. 16 September 2017; 3(1) Open Access. Published: 18 September 2017. doi: 10.23937/2572-4053.1510016.

27. Mills S., & Bone, K. (2000). *Principles and Practice of Phytotherapy: Modern Herbal Medicine.* Churchill Livingstone, London.

28. Srivastava, J. K., Shankar, E., & Gupta, S. (2010). Chamomile: A herbal medicine of the past with bright future. Mol Med Report. Author manuscript; available in PMC: 1 February 2011. Published in final edited form as: *Mol Med Report, 3*(6): 895–901.

29. Yang, R., Yuan, B. C., Ma, Y. S., Zhou, S., & Liu, Y. (2017). The anti-inflammatory activity of licorice, a widely used Chinese herb. *Pharm Biol*, 55(1): 5–18. E-pub: 21 September 2016.

30. Nurul, I. M., Mizuguchi, H., Shahriar, M., Venkatesh, P., Maeyama, K., Mukherjee, P. K., Hattori, M., Choudhuri, M. S., Takeda, N., & Fukui, H. (2011). Albizia lebbeck suppresses histamine signaling by the inhibition of histamine H1 receptor and histidine decarboxylase gene transcriptions. *Int Immunopharmacol*, 11(11): 1766–1772. E-pub: 2011 Jul 21. doi: 10.1016/j.intimp.2011.07.003.

31. Notes from Dr Lapraz: seminar on drainage.

32. Alonso, R., Cadavid, I., & Calleja, J. M. (1980). A preliminary study of hypoglycaemic activity of Rubus fruticosus. *Planta Med*, Suppl: 102–106.

33. Zia-Ul-Haq, M., Riaz, M., De Feo, V., & Jaafar, H. Z. E. (2014). Marius Review Rubus Fruticosus L.: Constituents, biological activities and health related uses. *Moga Molecules*, 19: 10998–11029. doi:10.3390/molecules190810998. Molecules ISSN 1420-3049. www.mdpi.com/journal/molecules.

34. Kumar, P., Kale, R. K., McLean, P., & Baquer, N. Z. (2012). Antidiabetic and neuroprotective effects of Trigonella foenum-graecum seed powder in diabetic rat brain. *Prague Med Rep*, 113(1): 33–43.

35. Lo, J.-M., Oliver, M. R., & Frulloni, L. (2013). Synopsis of recent guidelines on pancreatic exocrine insufficiency. *United European Gastroenterology Journal*, 1(2): 79–83. Reprints and permissions: sagepub.co.uk/journalsPermissions.nav. doi: 10.1177/2050640613476500 ueg.sagepub.com.

36. Notes from Dr Lapraz: seminar on pancreatic insufficiency.

37. Rathnavelu, V., Alitheen, N. B., Sohila, S., Kanagesan, S., & Ramesh, R. (2016). Potential role of bromelain in clinical and therapeutic applications. *Biomed Rep*, 5(3): 283–288. Published online: 18 July 2016. doi: 10.3892/br.2016.720 PMID: 27602208.

38. Sivaramakrishnan, G., & Sridharan, K. (2018). Role of serratiopeptidase after surgical removal of impacted molar: A systematic review and meta-analysis. *J Maxillofac Oral Surg*, 17(2): 122–128. Published online: 18 January 2017. doi: 10.1007/s12663-017-0996-9 PMID: 29618875.

39. Viswanatha Swamy, A. H. M., & Patil, P. A. (2008). Effect of some clinically used proteolytic enzymes on inflammation in rats. *Indian J Pharm Sci*, 70(1): 114–117. doi: 10.4103/0250-474X.40347.

40. Shah, D., & Mital, K. (2018). The role of trypsin: Chymotrypsin in tissue repair. *Adv Ther*, 35(1): 31–42. Published online: 5 December 2017. doi: 10.1007/s12325-017-0648-y.

41. Lapraz & Druaford: notes on Endobiogeny.

42. Lim, C. T., & Khoo, B. Endotext. Normal Physiology of ACTH and GH Release in the Hypothalamus and Anterior Pituitary in Man. Last Update: 24 October 2017.

43. Bertagna, X. (2017). Effects of chronic ACTH excess on human adrenal cortex. *Frontiers in endocrinology. Front Endocrinol (Lausanne)*, 8: 43. Published online: 8 March 2017. doi: 10.3389/fendo.2017.00043.

44. Raff, H., Sharma, S. T., & Nieman, L. K. (2014). Physiological basis for the etiology, diagnosis, and treatment of adrenal disorders: Cushing's Syndrome, adrenal insufficiency, and congenital adrenal hyperplasia. *Compr Physiol*, 4(2): 739–769. doi: 10.1002/cphy.c130035.

45. Higashi, S., & Aizawa, Y. (1980). Effect of ACTH on adrenal estrogens. *Jpn J Pharmacol*, *30*(3): 273–278.
46. Margioris, A. N., & Tsatsanis, C. Endotext. ACTH Action on the Adrenals. Last Update: 26 October 2016.
47. Talaber, G., Tuckermann, J. P., & Okret, S. *The FASEB journal*. ACTH controls thymocyte homeostasis independent of glucocorticoids. Published Online: 2 March 2015.
48. Celso, E. (2009). Gomez-Sanchez. Glucocorticoid production and regulation in thymus: Of mice and birds. *Endocrinology*, *150*(9): 3977–3979. doi: 10.1210/en. 2009-0615.
49. Johnson, E. W., Hughes, T. K., & Smith, E. M. (2005). ACTH enhancement of T-lymphocyte cytotoxic responses. *Cell Mol Neurobiol*, *25*(3–4): 743–757.
50. Hedayat & Lapraz. A clinical guide to applied systems biology. 2014: 84.
51. Chan, S., & Debono, M. (2010). Replication of cortisol circadian rhythm: new advances in hydrocortisone replacement therapy. *Ther Adv Endocrinol Metab*, *1*(3): 129–138. doi: 10.1177/2042018810380214.
52. Fauci, A. S., & Dale, D. C. (1974). The effect of in vivo hydrocortisone on subpopulations of human lymphocytes. *J Clin Invest*, *53*(1): 240–246.
53. Jefferies, W. M. (1991). Cortisol and immunity. *Med Hypotheses*, *34*(3): 198–208.
54. Mavoungou, E., Bouyou-Akotet, M. K., & Kremsner, P. G. (2005). Effects of prolactin and cortisol on natural killer (NK) cell surface expression and function of human natural cytotoxicity receptors (NKp46, NKp44 and NKp30). *Clin Exp Immunol*, *139*(2): 287–296.
55. Silverman, M. N., & Sternberg, E. M. (2012). Glucocorticoid regulation of inflammation and its behavioral and metabolic correlates: from HPA axis to glucocorticoid receptor dysfunction. *Ann N Y Acad Sci*. Author manuscript; available in PMC: 1 July 2013. Published in final edited form as: *Ann N Y Acad Sci*, *1261*: 55–63. doi: 10.1111/j.1749-6632.2012.06633.x.
56. Mawdsley, J. E., & Rampton, D. S. (2005). Psychological stress in IBD: new insights into pathogenic and therapeutic implications. *Gut*, *54*(10): 1481–1491.
57. Stasi, C., & Orlandelli, E. (2008). Role of the brain–gut axis in the pathophysiology of Crohn's disease. *Dig Dis*, *26*(2): 156–166. doi: 10.1159/000116774. E-pub: 21 April 2008.
58. Geer, E. B., Islam, J., & Buettner, C. (2014). Mechanisms of glucocorticoid-induced insulin resistance focus on adipose tissue function and lipid metabolism. *Endocrinol Metab Clin North Am*. Author manuscript; available in PMC: March 2015. Published in final edited form as: *Endocrinol Metab Clin North Am*, *43*(1): 75–102. doi: 10.1016/j. ecl.2013.10.005.
59. Kamba, A., Daimon, M., Murakami, H., Otaka, H., Matsuki, K., Sato, E., Tanabe, J., Takayasu, S., Matsuhashi, Y., Yanagimachi, M., Terui, K., Kageyama, K., Tokuda, I., Takahashi, I., & Nakaji, S. Association between higher serum cortisol levels and decreased insulin secretion in a general population. Published by *PLOS one*. Published: 18 November 2016.
60. Heyma, P., & Larkins, R. G. (1982). Glucocorticoids decrease in conversion of thyroxine into 3, 5, 3′-tri-iodothyronine by isolated rat renal tubules. *Clin Sci (Lond)*, *62*(2): 215–220.
61. Jia, D., O'Brien, C. A., Stewart, S. A., Manolagas, S. C., & Weinstein, R. S. (2006). Glucocorticoids act directly on osteoclasts to increase their life span and reduce bone density. Endocrinology. Author manuscript; available in PMC: 9 March 2007. Published

in final edited form as: *Endocrinology, 147*(12): 5592–5599. Published online: 24 August 2006. doi: 10.1210/en.2006-0459.

62. Canalis, E., & Delany, A. M. (2002). Mechanisms of glucocorticoid action in bone. *Ann N Y Acad Sci, 966*: 73–81.

63. Heisler, L. K., Pronchuk, N., Nonogaki, K., Zhou, L., Raber, J., Tung, L., Yeo, G. S., O'Rahilly, S., Colmers, W. F., Elmquist, J. K., & Tecott, L. H. (2007). Serotonin activates the hypothalamic-pituitary-adrenal axis via serotonin 2C receptor stimulation. *J Neurosci, 27*(26): 6956–6964.

64. Israelyan, N., & Margolis, K. G. (2019). Serotonin as a link between the gut-brain-microbiome axis in autism spectrum disorders. Pharmacol Res. Author manuscript; available in PMC: 7 February 2019. Published in final edited form as: *Pharmacol Res, 140*: 115–120. Published online: 15 January 2019. doi: 10.1016/j.phrs.2018.12.023.

65. Berger, M., Gray, J. A., & Roth, B. L. (2009). The expanded biology of serotonin. HHS Public Access Author Manuscript. *Annu Rev Med.* Author manuscript; available in PMC: 22 March 2018. Published in final edited form as: *Annu Rev Med, 60*: 355–366. doi:10.1146/annurev.med.60.042307.110802.

66. Chen, Q. Z., Zeng, Y. Z., Qu, Z. Q., Tang, T. Y., Qin, Y. J., Chung, P., Wong, R., & Hägg, U. (2009). The effects of Rhodiola rosea extract on 5-HT level, cell proliferation and quantity of neurons at cerebral hippocampus of depressive rats. *Phytomedicine, 16*(9): 830–888. E-pub: 28 April 2009. doi: 10.1016/j.phymed.2009.03.011.

67. Mannucci, C., Navarra, M., Calzavara, E., Caputi, A. P., & Calapai, G. (2012). Serotonin involvement in Rhodiola rosea attenuation of nicotine withdrawal signs in rats. *Phytomedicine, 19*(12): 1117–1124. E-pub: 24 August 2012. doi: 10.1016/j.phymed.2012.07.001.

68. Mao, J. J., Xie, S. X., Zee, J., Soeller, I., Li, Q. S., Rockwell, K., & Amsterdam, J. D. (2015). Rhodiola rosea versus sertraline for major depressive disorder: A randomized placebo-controlled trial. Phytomedicine. Author manuscript; available in PMC: 15 March 2016. Published in final edited form as: *Phytomedicine, 22*(3): 394–399. Published online: 23 February 2015. doi: 10.1016/j.phymed.2015.01.010.

69. Orlowski, M., & Sarao, M. S. Physiology, Follicle Stimulating Hormone. Last Update: 16 December 2018.

70. Lapraz & Durafford: notes on digestion.

71. Duraford & Lapraz: notes on gonadotrope axis.

72. Zirkin, B. R., & Papadopoulos, V. (2018). Review Leydig cells: formation, function, and regulation. *Biology of Reproduction, 99*(1): 101–111.

73. Carreau, S., Bouraima-Lelong, H., & Delalande, C. (2011). Estrogens in male germ cells. *Spermatogenesis, 1*(2): 90–94. doi: 10.4161/spmg.1.2.16766.

74. Barakat, R., Oakley, O., Kim, H., Jin, J., & Ko, C. J. (2016). Extra-gonadal sites of estrogen biosynthesis and function. *BMB Rep, 49*(9): 488–496. doi: 10.5483/BMBRep.2016.49.9.141.

75. Nelson, L. R., & Bulun, S. E. (2001). Estrogen production and action. *J Am Acad Dermatol, 45*(3 Suppl): S116–124.

76. Duraford & Lapraz: seminar notes on hepatitis.

77. Sapir-Koren, R., & Livshits, G. (2016). Rheumatoid arthritis onset in postmenopausal women: Does the ACPA seropositive subset result from genetic effects, estrogen deficiency, skewed profile of CD4(+) T-cells, and their interactions? *Mol Cell Endocrinol, 431*: 145–163. E-pub: 10 May 2016. doi: 10.1016/j.mce.2016.05.009.

78. Straub, R. H. (2007). The complex role of estrogens in inflammation. *Endocr Rev, 28*(5): 521–574. E-pub: 19 July 2007.
79. Kim, W.-U., Min, S.-Y., Hwang, S.-H., Yoo, S.-A., Kim, K. –J., & Cho, C.-S. (2010). Effect of oestrogen on T-cell apoptosis in patients with systemic lupus erythematosus. *Clin Exp Immunol, 161*(3): 453–458. doi: 10.1111/j.1365-2249.2010.04194.x.
80. Mok, C. C., & Lau, C. S. (2003). Pathogenesis of systemic lupus erythematosus. *J Clin Pathol, 56*(7): 481–490. doi: 10.1136/jcp.56.7.481.
81. Alpízar-Rodríguez, D., Pluchino, N., Canny, G., Gabay, C., & Finckh, A. (2017). The role of female hormonal factors in the development of rheumatoid arthritis. *Rheumatology, 56*(8): 1254–1263. doi: 10.1093/rheumatology/kew318.
82. Pierdominici, M., Maselli, A., Varano, B., Barbati, C., Cesaro, P., Spada, C., Zullo, A., Lorenzetti, R., Rosati, M., Rainaldi, G., Limiti, M. R., Guidi, L., Conti, L., & Oncotarget, S. G. (2015). Linking estrogen receptor β expression with inflammatory bowel disease activity. 6(38): 40443–40451. Published online 2015 Oct 22. doi: 10.18632/oncotarget.6217.
83. Langen, L-v., Hotte, N., Dieleman, L. A., Albert, E., Mulder, C., & Madsen, K. L. (2011). Estrogen receptor-β signaling modulates epithelial barrier function. *Am J Physiol Gastrointest Liver Physiol, 300*(4): G621–26. E-pub: 20 January 2011.doi: 10.1152/ajpgi.00274.2010.
84. Gardner, D. G., & Shoback, D. (2007). *Greenspan's Basic & Clinical Endocrinology.* Eighth edition. McGraw-Hill Medical. 121.
85. Antoniou-Tsigkos, A., Zapanti, E., Ghizzoni, L., & Mastorakos, G. Endotext. Adrenal Androgens. Created: 5 January 2019.
86. Balfour, W. E., Comline, R. S., & Short, R. V. (1957). Secretion of Progesterone by the Adrenal Gland. *Nature International Journal of Science, 180*: 1480–1481.
87. Oettel, M., & Mukhopadhyay, A. K. (2004). Progesterone: the forgotten hormone in men? *Aging Male, 7*(3): 236–257.
88. Ranelletti, F. O., Piantelli, M., Zanella, E., Capelli, A., & Farinon, A. M. Hepatology. Estrogen and progesterone receptors in the gallbladders from patients with gallstones. First published: October 1991.
89. Malini, T., Vanithakumari, G., Megala, N., Anusya, S., Devi, K., & Elango, V. (1985). Effect of Foeniculum vulgare Mill. seed extract on the genital organs of male and female rats. *Indian J Physiol Pharmacol, 29*(1): 21–26.
90. Notes from Lapraz: seminar on thyrotropic axis.
91. Breese, G. R., Mueller, R. A., Mailman, R. B., & Frye, G. D. (1981). Effects of TRH on central nervous system function. *Prog Clin Biol Res, 68*: 99–116.
92. Campbell, M., & Jialal, I. Physiology, Endocrine Hormones. Author Information. Last Update: 23 February 2019.
93. Loosen, P. T. (1985). The TRH-induced TSH response in psychiatric patients: a possible neuroendocrine marker. *Psychoneuroendocrinology, 10*(3): 237–260.
94. Wolkin, A., Peselow, E. D., Smith, M., Lautin, A., Kahn, I., & Rotrosen, J. (1984). TRH test abnormalities in psychiatric disorders. *J Affect Disord, 6*(3–4): 273–281.
95. Štrbák, V. (2018). Pancreatic Thyrotropin Releasing Hormone and Mechanism of Insulin Secretion. *Cell Physiol Biochem, 50*(1): 378–384. E-pub: 4 October 2018. doi: 10.1159/000494013.

96. Benický, J., & Štrbák, V. (2000). Glucose stimulates and insulin inhibits release of pancreatic TRH in vitro. *Eur J Endocrinol, 142*(1): 60–65.

97. Dutton, C. M., Joba, W., Spitzweg, C., Heufelder, A. E., & Bahn, R. S. (1997). Thyrotropin receptor expression in adrenal, kidney, and thymus. *Thyroid, 7*(6): 879–884.

98. Tuchendler, D., & Bolanowski, M. (2014). The influence of thyroid dysfunction on bone metabolism. *Thyroid Res, 7*: 12. Published online: 20 December 2014. doi: 10.1186/s13044-014-0012-0.

99. Mancini, A., Di Segni, C., Raimondo, S., Olivieri, G., Silvestrini, A., Meucci, E., & Currò, D. Thyroid Hormones, Oxidative Stress, and Inflammation. Hindawi Publishing Corporation Mediators of Inflammation. 2016; Article ID 6757154: 12.

100. van der Spek, A. H., Fliers, E., & Boelen, A. (2017). Thyroid hormone metabolism in innate immune cells. *Journal of Endocrinology, 232*: R67–R81.

101. Hodkinson, C. V., Simpson, E. E., Beattie, J. H., O'Connor, J. M., Campbell, D. J., Strain, J. J., & Wallace, J. M. (2009). Preliminary evidence of immune function modulation by thyroid hormones in healthy men and women aged 55–70 years. *J Endocrinol, 202*(1): 55–63. E-pub: 27 April 2009. doi: 10.1677/JOE-08-0488.

102. Jara, E. L., Muñoz-Durango, N., Llanos, C., Fardella, C., González, P. A., Bueno, S. M., Kalergis, A. M., & Riedel, C. A. (2017). Modulating the function of the immune system by thyroid hormones and thyrotropin. *Immunol Lett, 184*: 76–83. E-pub: 17 February 2017. doi: 10.1016/j.imlet.2017.02.010.

103. Beer, A. M., Wiebelitz, K. R., & Schmidt-Gayk, H. (2008). Lycopus europaeus (Gypsywort): effects on the thyroidal parameters and symptoms associated with thyroid function. *Phytomedicine, 15*(1–2): 16–22.

104. Yarnell, E., & Abascal, K. (2006). Botanical medicine for thyroid regulation. *Alternative and Complementary Therapies, 12*(3). Published Online: 12 June 2006. doi: 10.1089/act.2006.12.107.

105. Santini, F., Vitti, P., Ceccarini, G., Mammoli, C., Rosellini, V., Pelosini, C., Marsili, A., Tonacchera, M., Agretti, P., Santoni, T., Chiovato, L., & Pinchera, A. (2003). In vitro assay of thyroid disruptors affecting TSH-stimulated adenylate cyclase activity. *J Endocrinol Invest, 26*(10): 950–955.

106. Durraford & Lapraz: notes on somatotropic axis.

107. Giustina, A., Mazziotti, G., & Canalis, E. (2008). Growth hormone, insulin-like growth factors, and the skeleton. *Endocrine Reviews, 29*(5): 535–559. doi: 10.1210/er.2007-0036.

108. Kim, S.-H., & Park, M.-J. (2017). Effects of growth hormone on glucose metabolism and insulin resistance in human. *Ann Pediatr Endocrinol Metab, 22*(3): 145–152. Published online: 28 September 2017. doi: 10.6065/apem.2017. 22.3.145.

109. Inoue, Y., Copeland, E. M., & Souba, W. W. (1994). Growth hormone enhances amino acid uptake by the human small intestine. *Ann Surg, 219*(6): 715–724.

110. Bjøro, T., Ostberg, B. C., Sand, O., Torjesen, P. A., Penman, E., Gordeladze, J. O., Iversen, J. G., Gautvik, K. M., & Haug, E. (1988). Somatostatin inhibits prolactin secretion by multiple mechanisms involving a site of action distal to increased cyclic adenosine 3′,5′-monophosphate and elevated cytosolic Ca2+ in rat lactotrophs. *Acta Physiol Scand, 133*(3): 271–282.

111. Fitzgerald, P., & Dinan, T. G. (2008). Prolactin and dopamine: what is the connection? A review article. *J Psychopharmacol, 22*(2 Suppl): 12–9.

112. Al-Chalabi, M., & Alsalman, I. Physiology, Prolactin. Author Information. Last Update: 16 April 16 2019.

113. Borba, V. V., Zandman-Goddard, G., & Shoenfeld, Y. Prolactin and Autoimmunity. *Front. Immunol.* 12 February 2018.

114. Díaz, L., Muñoz, M. D., González, L., Lira-Albarrán, S., Larrea, F., & Méndez, I. Prolactin in the Immune System. Open access peer-reviewed chapter. Submitted: 5 December 2011. Reviewed: 24 September 2012. Published: 23 January 2013. doi: 10.5772/53538.

115. Mok, C. C., & C. S. (2003). Pathogenesis of systemic lupus erythematosus. *Lau. J Clin Pathol*, 56(7): 481–490. doi: 10.1136/jcp.56.7.481.

116. Wu, W., Sun, M., Zhang, H. P., Chen, T., Wu, R., Liu, C., Yang, G., Geng, X R., Feng, B. S., Liu, Z., Liu, Z., & Yang, P. C. (2014). Prolactin mediates psychological stress-induced dysfunction of regulatory T-cells to facilitate intestinal inflammation. *Gut*, 63(12): 1883–1892. E-pub: 18 February 2014.

117. Park, S., Kang, S., Lee, H. W., & Bo, K. S. (2012). Central prolactin modulates insulin sensitivity and insulin secretion in diabetic rats. *Neuroendocrinology*, 95(4): 332–343. E-pub: 21 March 2012. doi: 10.1159/000336501.

118. Song, G., Pacini, G., Ahrén, B., & D'Argenio, D. Z. (2017). Peptides. Glucagon increases insulin levels by stimulating insulin secretion without effect on insulin clearance in mice. Author manuscript; available in PMC: 1 February 2018. Published in final edited form as: Peptides. February 2017; 88: 74–79. Published online: 21 December 2016. doi: 10.1016/j.peptides.2016.12.012.

119. De Felice, F. G., Lourenco, M. V., & Ferreira, S. T. (2014). How does brain insulin resistance develop in Alzheimer's disease? *Alzheimer's Dement*, 10(1 Suppl): S26–32. doi: 10.1016/j.jalz.2013.12.004.

120. Ceolotto, G., Bevilacqua, M., Papparella, I., Baritono, E., Franco, L., Corvaja, C., Mazzoni, M., Semplicini, A., & Avogaro, A. (2004). Insulin generates free radicals by an NAD(P)H, Phosphatidylinositol 3′-Kinase-dependent mechanism in human skin fibroblasts ex vivo. *Diabetes*, 53(5): 1344–1351.

121. Giacco, F., & Brownlee, M. (2010). Oxidative stress and diabetic complications. *Circ Res.* Author manuscript; available in PMC: 29 October 2011. Published in final edited form as: *Circ Res*, 107(9): 1058–1070. doi: 10.1161/CIRCRESAHA.110.223545.

122. Kumar, D., Shankar, K., Patel, S., Gupta, A., Varshney, S., Gupta, S., Rajan, S., Srivastava, A., Vishwakarma, A. L., & Gaikwad, A. N. (2018). Chronic hyperinsulinemia promotes meta-inflammation and extracellular matrix deposition in adipose tissue: Implications of nitric oxide. *Mol Cell Endocrinol*, 477: 15–28. doi: 10.1016/j.mce.2018.05.010. E-pub: 10 May 2018.

123. Crofts, C. A. P., Zinn, C., Wheldon, M. C., & Schofield, G. M. (2015). Hyperinsulinemia: A unifying theory of chronic disease? *Diabesity*, 1(4): 34–43. doi: 10.15562/diabesity.2015.19 www.diabesity.ejournals.ca.

124. Dinan, T. G., Stilling, R. M., Stanton, C., & Cryan, J. F. (2015). Collective unconscious: how gut microbes shape human behavior. *J Psychiatr Res*, 63: 1–9. E-pub: 3 March 2015. doi: 10.1016/j.jpsychires.2015.02.021.

125. Messaoudi, M., Violle, N., Bisson, J.-F., Desor, D., Javelot, H., & Rougeot, C. (2011). Beneficial psychological effects of a probiotic formulation (*Lactobacillus helveticus* R0052 and *Bifidobacterium longum* R0175) in healthy human volunteers. *Gut Microbes*, 2(4): 256–261, Received: 20 April 2011. Accepted: 21 Jul 2011. Published online: 1 Jul 2011.

126. Cecchini, D. A., Laville, E., Laguerre, S., Robe, P., Leclerc, M., Doré, J., Henrissat, B., Remaud-Siméon, M., Monsan, P., & Potocki-Véronèse, G. (2013). Functional metagenomics reveals novel pathways of prebiotic breakdown by human gut bacteria. *PLOS one, 8*(9): e72766. eCollection 2013. doi: 10.1371/journal.pone.0072766.

127. Dunn, A. B., Jordan, S., Baker, B. J., & Carlson, N. S. (2017). The Maternal Infant Microbiome: Considerations for Labour and Birth. *MCN Am J Matern Child Nurs.* 1 November 2018. Published in final edited form as: *MCN Am J Matern Child Nurs, 42*(6): 318–325.

128. Rea, K., Dinanab, T. G., & Cryanac, J. F. (2016). The microbiome: A key regulator of stress and neuroinflammation. Author links open overlay panel. *Neurobiology of Stress, 4*: 23–33.

129. Gevers, D., Kugathasan, S., Denson, L. A., Huttenhower, C., Knight, R., & Xavier, R. J. (2014). The treatment-naive microbiome in new-onset Crohn's disease. *Cell host and microbe. Resource, 15*(3): 382–392.

130. Krishnan, A. N. A., Luo, C., Yajnik, V., Khalili, H., Garber, J. J., Stevens, B. W., Cleland, T., & Xavier, R. J. (2017). Gut microbiome function predicts response to anti-integrin biologic therapy in inflammatory bowel diseases. *Cell host and microbe, 21*(5): 603–610.

131. Gevers, D., Kugathasan, S., Knights, D., Kostic, A. D., Knight, R., & Xavier, R. J. (2017). A microbiome foundation for the study of Crohn's disease. Elsevier. *Cell Host & Microbe, 21.* doi: 10.1016/j.chom.2017.02.012/.

132. Evans, J. M., Morris, L. S., & Marchesi, J. R. (2013). The gut microbiome: the role of a virtual organ in the endocrinology of the host. Role of a virtual organ in host endocrinology. *Society for Endocrinology, 218*(3): R37–R47.

133. Cianci, R., Pagliari, D., Piccirillo, C. A., Fritz, J. H., & Gambassi, G. The Microbiota and Immune System Crosstalk in Health and Disease. Hindawi Mediators of Inflammation. 2018; Article ID 2912539: 3. doi: 10.1155/2018/2912539.

134. Russell, W. R., Hoyles, L., Flint, H. J., & Dumas, M. E. (2013). Colonic bacterial metabolites and human health. *Curr Opin Microbiol, 16*(3): 246–254.

135. Schmitz, H., Fromm, M., Bentzel, C. J., Scholz, P., Detjen, K., Mankertz, J., Bode, H., Epple, H. J., Riecken, E. O., & Schulzke, J. D. (1999). Tumor necrosis factor-alpha (TNFalpha) regulates the epithelial barrier in the human intestinal cell line HT-29/B6. *J Cell Sci, 112* (Pt 1): 137–146.

136. Spiller, R., Aziz, Q., Creed, F., Emmanuel, A., Houghton, L., Hungin, P., Jones, R., Kumar, D., Rubin, G., Trudgill, N., & Whorwell, P. (2007). Guidelines on the irritable bowel syndrome: mechanisms and practical management. Clinical Services Committee of The British Society of Gastroenterology. *Gut, 56*(12): 1770–1798. E-pub: 8 May 2007.

137. Pusceddu, M. M., Murray, K., & Gareau, M. G. (2018). Targeting the microbiota, from irritable bowel syndrome to mood disorders: Focus on probiotics and prebiotics. *Curr Pathobiol Rep, 6*(1): 1–13. Published online: 12 February 2018. doi: 10.1007/s40139-018-0160-3.

138. Drew, P. D., & Chavis, J. A. (2000). Inhibition of microglial cell activation by cortisol. *Brain Res Bull, 52*(5): 391–396.

139. Wohleb, E. S., McKim, D. B., Sheridan, J. F., & Godbout, J. P. (2014). Monocyte trafficking to the brain with stress and inflammation: a novel axis of immune-to-brain communication that influences mood and behaviour. *Front Neurosci, 8*: 447. Published online: 21 January 2015.

140. Chavan, R. S., Pannaraj, P. S., Luna, R. A., Szabo, S., Adesina, A., Versalovic, J., Krance, R. A., & Kennedy-Nasser, A. A. (2013). Significant morbidity and mortality attributable to rothia mucilaginosa infections in children with hematological malignancies or following hematopoietic stem cell transplantation. *Pediatr Hematol Oncol, 30*(5): 445–454. 9 May 2013.

141. Becker, C., Neurath, M. F., & Wirtz, S. (2015). The intestinal microbiota in inflammatory bowel disease. *ILAR J, 56*(2): 192–204. doi: 10.1093/ilar/ilv030.

142. Forbes, J. D., Domselaar, G. V., & Bernstein, C. N. (2016). The gut microbiota in immune-mediated inflammatory diseases. *Front Microbiol, 7*: 1081. Published online: 11 July 2016.

143. Knights, D., Silverberg, M. S., Weersma, R. K., Gevers, D., Dijkstra, G., Huang, H., Tyler, A. D., Sommeren, S.-v., Imhann, F., Stempak, J. M., Huang, H., Vangay, P., Al-Ghalith, G. A., Russell, C., Sauk, J., Knight, J., Daly, M. J., Huttenhower, C., & Xavier, R. J. (2014). Complex host genetics influence the microbiome in inflammatory bowel disease. *Genome Medicinevolume, 6*, Article number: 107.

144. Kostic, A. D., Xavier, R. J., & Gevers, D. (2014). The microbiome in inflammatory bowel disease: current status and the future ahead. *Gastroenterology, 146*(6): 1489–1499. E-pub: 19 February 2014.

145. Rivière, A., Selak, M., Lantin, D., Leroy, F., & De Vuyst, L. (2016). Bifidobacteria and butyrate-producing colon bacteria: importance and strategies for their stimulation in the human gut. *Front Microbiol, 7*: 979. Published online: 2016 Jun 28.

146. Jostins, L., et al. (2012). Host-microbe interactions have shaped the genetic architecture of inflammatory bowel disease. Nature. Author manuscript. Available in PMC: 2013 May 1. Published in final edited form as: *Nature, 491*(7422): 119–124.

147. O'Mahony, S. M., Clarke, G., Dinan, T. G., & Cryan, J. F. (2017). Early-life adversity and brain development: Is the microbiome a missing piece of the puzzle?. *Neuroscience, 342*: 37–54. E-pub: 2015 Oct 1. doi: 10.1016/j.neuroscience.2015.09.068.

148. Borre, Y., O'Keeffe, G. W., Clarke, G., Stanton, C., Dinan, T. G., & Cryan, J. F. (2014). Microbiota and neurodevelopmental windows: implications for brain disorders. *Trends Mol Med, 20*(9): 509–518. E-pub: 20 June 2014. doi: 10.1016/j.molmed.2014.05.002.

149. Vučic', D. M., Petkovic', M. R., Rodic'-Grabovac, B. B., Stefanovic', O. D., Vasic', S. M., & Čomic', L. R. (2013). *Advanced Research Journal of Microbiology, 1*(4): 67–073.

150. Thanina, A. C., Mourad, B., & Karim, A. (2015). Antibacterial activity of two extracts from Rubus fruticosus L. against resistant pathogens and their antioxidant potential. *African Journal of Microbiology Research, 9*(18): 1255–1262, doi: 10.5897/AJMR2015.7437 Article Number: BC5124653178 ISSN 1996-0808.

151. Alkhawajah, A. M. (1997). Studies on the antimicrobial activity of juglans regia. *Am J Chin Med, 25*(2): 175–180.

152. Pereira, J. A., Oliveira, I., Sousa, A., Valentão, P., Andrade, P. B., Ferreira, I. C., Ferreres, F., Bento, A., Seabra, R., & Estevinho, L. (2007). Walnut (*Juglans regia* L.) leaves: phenolic compounds, antibacterial activity and antioxidant potential of different cultivars. *Food Chem Toxicol, 45*(11): 2287–2295. E-pub: 12 June 2007.

153. Saeed, S., & Tariq, P. (2009). Antibacterial activity of oregano (Origanum vulgare Linn.) against gram positive bacteria. *Pak J Pharm Sci, 22*(4): 421–424.

154. Boughendjioua, H., & Seridi, R. (2017). Antimicrobial efficacy of the essential oil of origanum vulgare from Algeria. *Journal of Pharmacy and Pharmacology Research*, ISSN: 2578-1553.

155. Karuppiah, P., & Rajaram, S. (2012). Antibacterial effect of Allium sativum cloves and Zingiber officinale rhizomes against multiple-drug resistant clinical pathogens. *Asian Pac J Trop Biomed*, 2(8): 597–601. doi: 10.1016/S2221-1691(12)60104-X.

156. Abiy, E., & Berhe, A. (2016). Anti-bacterial effect of garlic (Allium sativum) against clinical isolates of staphylococcus aureus and escherichia coli from patients attending hawassa referral hospital, Ethiopia. Published date: 14 November 2016. *J Infec Dis Treat*, 2:2. doi:10.21767/2472-1093.100023.

157. Nabavi, S. F., Di Lorenzo, A., Izadi, M., Sobarzo-Sánchez, E., Daglia, M., & Nabavi, S. M. (2015). Antibacterial effects of cinnamon: From farm to food, cosmetic and pharmaceutical industries. *Nutrients*, 7(9): 7729–7748. Published online: 11 September 2015.

158. Wanga, Y., Zhang, Y., Shia, Y.-q., Pana, X.-h., Lu, Y.-h., & Cao, R. (2018). Antibacterial effects of cinnamon (Cinnamomum zeylanicum) bark essential oil on Porphyromonas gingivalis. *Microbial Pathogenesis*, 116: 26–32.

159. Heghes, S. C., Vostinaru, O., Rus, L. M., Mogosan, C., Iuga, C. A., & Filip, L. (2019). Antispasmodic effect of essential oils and their constituents: A review. *Molecules*, 24(9): 1675. Published online: 2019 Apr 29. doi: 10.3390/molecules24091675.

160. Badgujar, S. B., Patel, V. V., & Bandivdekar, A. H. (2014). Foeniculum vulgare Mill: A review of its botany, phytochemistry, pharmacology, contemporary application, and toxicology. *Biomed Res Int*, 2014: 842674. Published online: 3 August 2014. doi: 10.1155/2014/842674.

161. Yang, L., Chai, C. Z., Yan, Y., Duan, Y. D., Henz, A., Zhang, B. L., Backlund, A., Yu, B. Y. (2017). Spasmolytic mechanism of aqueous licorice extract on oxytocin-induced uterine. Contraction through inhibiting the phosphorylation of heat shock protein 27. *Molecules*, 22(9): pii: E1392. doi: 10.3390/molecules22091392.

162. Khalaj, A., & Khani, S. (2018). Spasmolytic effects of hydroalcoholic extract of Melissa officinalis on isolated rat ileum. *Journal of reports in pharmaceutical sciences* 7(3): 260–269.

163. Johri, R. K. (2011). Cuminum cyminum and Carum carvi. *Pharmacogn Rev*, 5(9): 63–72. doi: 10.4103/0973-7847.79101.

164. Mehmood, M. H., corresponding author: Munir, S., Khalid, U. A., Asrar, M., & Gilani, A. H.,. Antidiarrhoeal, antisecretory and antispasmodic activities of Matricaria chamomilla are mediated predominantly through K+-channels activation. *BMC Complement Altern Med*, 15: 75. Published online: 24 March 2015. doi: 10.1186/s12906-015-0595-6.

165. Yazdi, H., Seifi, A., Changizi, S., Khori, V., Hossini, F., Davarian, A., Jand, Y., Enayati, A., Mazandarani, M., & Nanvabashi, F. (2017). Hydro-alcoholic extract of Matricaria recutita exhibited dual antispasmodic effect via modulation of Ca2+ channels, NO and PKA2-kinase pathway in rabbit jejunum. *Avicenna J Phytomed*, 7(4): 334–344.

166. Kianpour, M., Mansouri, A., Mehrabi, T., & Asghari, G. (2016). Effect of lavender scent inhalation on prevention of stress, anxiety and depression in the postpartum period. *Iran J Nurs Midwifery Res*, 21(2): 197–201. doi: 10.4103/1735-9066.178248.

167. Andrew Chavalier. Encyclopedia of herbs.

168. Beheshti-Rouy, M., Azarsina, M., Rezaie-Soufi, L., Alikhani, M. Y., Roshanaie, G., & Komaki, S. (2015). The antibacterial effect of sage extract (Salvia officinalis) mouthwash against Streptococcus mutans in dental plaque: a randomized clinical trial. *Iran J Microbiol*, 7(3): 173–177.

169. Gericke, S., Lübken, O. T., Wolf, O. D., Kaiser, M., Hannig, C., & Speer, K. (2018). Identification of new compounds from sage flowers (Salvia officinalis L.) as markers for quality control and the influence of the manufacturing technology on the chemical composition and antibacterial activity of sage flower extracts. *J. Agric. Food Chem*, *668*: 1843–1853. Publication Date: 16 February 2018.

170. Alexa, E., Sumalan, R. M., Danciu, C., Obistioiu, D., Negrea, M., Poiana, M.-A., Rus, C., Radulov, I., Pop, G., & Dehelean, C. (2018). Synergistic anti-fungal, allelopatic and anti-proliferative potential of Salvia officinalis L., and Thymus vulgaris L. essential oils. *Molecules*, *23*(1): 185. Published online: 16 January 2018. doi: 10.3390/molecules23010185.

171. Pinto, E., Vale-Silva, L., Cavaleiro, C., & Salgueiro, L. (2009). Anti-fungal activity of the clove essential oil from Syzygium aromaticum on Candida, Aspergillus and dermatophyte species. *Journal of Medical Microbiology*, *58*: 1454–1462.

172. de Lira Mota, K. S., de Oliveira Pereira, F., de Oliveira, W. A., Lima, I. O., de Oliveira Lima, E. (2012). Anti-fungal activity of Thymus vulgaris L. essential oil and its constituent phytochemicals against Rhizopus oryzae: interaction with ergosterol. *Molecules*, *17*(12): 14418–14433. doi: 10.3390/molecules171214418.

173. Čabarkapa, I., Čolovic', R., Đuragic', O., Popovic', S., Kokic', B., Milanov, D., & Pezo, L. (2019). Anti-biofilm activities of essential oils rich in carvacrol and thymol against Salmonella Enteritidis. *Biofouling*, *35*(3): 361–375. E-pub: 14 May 2019. doi: 10.1080/08927014.2019.1610169.

174. Pereira, J. A., Oliveira, I., Sousa, A., Valentão, P., Andrade, P. B., Ferreira, I. C. F. R., Ferreres, F., Bento, A., Seabra, R., & Estevinho, L. (2007). Food and Chemical Toxicology. Walnut (Juglans regia L.) leaves: Phenolic compounds, antibacterial activity and antioxidant potential of different cultivars. *Elsevier. Food and Chemical Toxicology*, *45*(11): 2287–2295.

175. Wang, Y., Zhang, Y., Shi, Y. Q., Pan, X. H., Lu, Y. H., & Cao, P. (2018). Antibacterial effects of cinnamon (Cinnamomum zeylanicum) bark essential oil on Porphyromonas gingivalis. *Microb Pathog*, *116*: 26–32 E-pub: 9 January 2018. doi: 10.1016/j.micpath.2018.01.009.

176. Firmino, D. F., Cavalcante, T. T. A., Gomes, G. A., Firmino, N. C. S., Rosa, L. D., de Carvalho, M. G., & Catunda, F. E. A. Jr., (2018). Antibacterial and Antibiofilm Activities of Cinnamomum sp. Essential Oil and Cinnamaldehyde: Antimicrobial Activities. The Scientific World Journal, Article ID 7405736: 9.

177. Yap, Y. A., & Mariño, E. (2018). An insight into the intestinal web of mucosal immunity, microbiota, and diet in inflammation. Front Immunol, 9: 2617. Published online: 20 November 2018. doi: 10.3389/fimmu.2018.02617.

178. Shi, N., Li, N., Duan, X., & Niucorresponding, H. (2017). Interaction between the gut microbiome and mucosal immune system. Mil Med Res, 4: 14. Published online: 27 April 2017.

179. Marchiando, A. M., Graham, W. V., & Turner, J. R. (2010). Epithelial barriers in homeostasis and disease. *Annu Rev Pathol*, *5*: 119–144. doi: 10.1146/annurev.pathol.4.110807.092135.

180. Kuhn, K. A., Pedraza, I., & Demoruelle, M. K. (2014). Mucosal immune responses to microbiota in the development of autoimmune disease. *Rheum Dis Clin North Am*, *40*(4): 711–725. E-pub: 4 September 2014 Sep 4.

181. Seksik, P., Rigottier-Gois, L., Gramet, G., Sutren, M., Pochart, P., Marteau, P., Jian, R., & Doré, J. (2003). Alterations of the dominant faecal bacterial groups in patients with Crohn's disease of the colon. *Gut*, *52*(2): 237–242. doi: 10.1136/gut.52.2.237.

182. Spehlmann, M. E., Begun, A. Z., Burghardt, J., Lepage, P., Raedler, A., & Schreiber, S. (2008). Epidemiology of inflammatory bowel disease in a German twin cohort: results of a nationwide study. *Inflamm Bowel Dis*, *14*(7): 968–976.

183. Visser, J., Rozing, J., Sapone, A., Lammers, K., & Fasanob, A. (2009). Tight junctions, intestinal permeability, and autoimmunity celiac disease and type 1 diabetes paradigms. *Ann N Y Acad Sci, 1165*: 195–205. doi: 10.1111/j. 1749-6632.2009.04037.x

184. Notes from Dr Lapraz: seminar on microbiome.

185. Notes from Dr Lapraz: seminar on IBS and IBD.

186. Saha, L. Irritable bowel syndrome: Pathogenesis, diagnosis, treatment, and evidence-based medicine. *World J Gastroenterol, 20*(22): 6759–6773. Published online: 14 Jun 2014. doi: 10.3748/wjg.v20.i22.6759.

187. Soares, R. L. S. (2014). Irritable bowel syndrome: A clinical review. *World J Gastroenterol, 20*(34): 12144–12160. Published online: 14 September 2014.

188. Occhipinti, K., & Smith, J. W. (2012). Irritable bowel syndrome: A review and update. *Clin Colon Rectal Surg, 25*(1): 46–52.

189. Ng, S. C., Shi, H. Y., Hamidi, N., Underwood, F. E., Tang, W., Benchimol, E. I., Panaccione, R., Ghosh, S., Wu, J. C. Y., Chan, F. K. L., Sung, J. J. Y. & Kaplan, G. G. (2018). Worldwide incidence and prevalence of inflammatory bowel disease in the 21st century: a systematic review of population-based studies. *Lancet, 390*(10114): 2769–2778. E-pub: 16 October 2017. doi: 10.1016/S0140-6736(17)32448-0.

190. Boyapati, R., Satsangi, J., & Ho, G. T. (2015). Pathogenesis of Crohn's disease. F1000Prime Rep, 7: 44. Published online: 2 April 2015. doi: 10.12703/P7-44.

191. Abraham, C., & Cho, J. H. (2009). Inflammatory bowel disease. *N Engl J Med, 361*(21): 2066–2078. doi: 10.1056/NEJMra0804647.

192. Walfish, A. E., & Companioni, R. A. C. MSD MANUAL Professional Version. Ulcerative Colitis By Aaron E. Walfish, MD, Mount Sinai Medical Center; Rafael Antonio Ching Companioni, MD, Icahn School of Medicine, Elmhurst Hospital Center. Last full review/revision April 2019 by https://www.msdmanuals.com/en-gb/professional/gastrointestinal-disorders/inflammatory-bowel-disease-ibd/ulcerative-colitis.

193. https://www.mayoclinic.org/diseases-conditions/inflammatory-bowel-disease/symptoms-causes/syc-20353315. Mayo clinic. Inflammatory bowel disease.

194. Lapraz, J. C., & Hedayat, K. M. (2013). Global advances in health and medicine. Endobiogeny: A Global Approach to Systems Biology (part 1 of 2). 2(1).

195. Notes from Dr Lapraz: seminar on functional biology.

196. Wilson, M. J. (2003). Clay mineralogical and related characteristics of geophagic materials. *J Chem Ecol*, *29*(7): 1525–1547.

197. Jacob, A., Wu, R., Zhou, M., & Wang, P. (2007). Mechanism of the anti-inflammatory effect of curcumin: PPAR-g activation. PPAR Res, 2007: 89369. Published online: 17 January 2008. doi: 10.1155/2007/89369.

198. Jurenka, J. S. (2009). Anti-inflammatory properties of curcumin, a major constituent of Curcuma longa: a review of preclinical and clinical research. *Altern Med Rev, 14*(2): 141–153.

199. Bagad, A. S., Joseph, J. A., Bhaskaran, N., & Agarwal, A. (2013). Research Article. Comparative Evaluation of Anti-Inflammatory Activity of Curcuminoids, Turmerones, and Aqueous Extract of Curcuma longa. Advances in Pharmacological Sciences, Article ID 805756: 7. http://dx.doi.org/10.1155/ 2013/805756.

200. Catanzaro, D., Rancan, S., Orso, G., Dall'Acqua, S., Brun, P., Giron, M. C., Carrara, M., Castagliuolo, I., Ragazzi, E., Caparrotta, L., & Montopoli, M. (2015). Boswellia serrata preserves intestinal epithelial barrier from oxidative and inflammatory damage. PLOS One. 10(5): e0125375. Published online: 8 May 2015. doi: 10.1371/journal.pone.0125375.

201. Siddiqui M. Z., & Serrata, B. (2011). A potential anti-inflammatory agent: An overview. Indian J Pharm Sci, 73(3): 255–261. doi: 10.4103/0250-474X.93507.

202. Bertocchi, M., Isani, G., Medici, F., Andreani, G., Usca, I. T., Roncada, P., Forni, M., & Bernardini, C. (2018). Anti-inflammatory activity of Boswellia serrata extracts: An in vitro study on porcine aortic endothelial cells. Oxid Med Cell Longev, 2018: 2504305. Published online: 25 June 2018. doi: 10.1155/2018/2504305.

203. Frattaruolo, L., Carullo, G., Brindisi, M., Mazzotta, S., Bellissimo, L., Rago, V., Curcio, R., Dolce, V., Aiello, F., & Cappello, A. R. (2019). Antioxidant and Anti-Inflammatory Activities of Flavanones from Glycyrrhiza glabra L. (licorice) Leaf Phytocomplexes: Identification of Licoflavanone as a Modulator of NF-κB/MAPK Pathway. Antioxidants (Basel), 8(6): 186. Published online: 20 June 2019. doi: 10.3390/antiox8060186.

204. Yang, R., Yuan, B. C., Ma, Y. S., Zhou, S., & Liu, Y. The anti-inflammatory activity of licorice, a widely used Chinese herb, ages 5–18. Journal of Pharmaceutical Biology, 55(1). Received: 30 Jul 2015. Accepted 13 Aug 2016. Published online: 21 Sep 2016.

205. Ettefagh, K. A., Burns, J. T., Junio, H. A., Kaatz, G. W., & Cech, N. B. (2011). Goldenseal (Hydrastis canadensis L.) extracts synergistically enhance the antibacterial activity of berberine via efflux pump inhibition. Planta Med. Author manuscript; available in PMC: 24 May 2011. Published in final edited form as: Planta Med, 77(8): 835–840. Published online 14 December 2010. doi: 10.1055/s-0030-1250606.

206. Garbacki, N., Tits, M., Angenot, L., & Damas, J. (2004). Inhibitory effects of proanthocyanidins from Ribes nigrum leaves on carrageenin acute inflammatory reactions induced in rats. BMC Pharmacol, 4: 25.

207. Lee, Y., & Lee, J. Y. (2019). Blackcurrant (Ribes nigrum) Extract Exerts an Anti-Inflammatory Action by Modulating Macrophage Phenotypes. Nutrients. 11(5). pii: E975. doi: 10.3390/nu11050975.

208. Garbacki, N., Kinet, M., Nusgens, B., Desmecht, D., Damas, J. (2005). Proanthocyanidins, from Ribes nigrum leaves, reduce endothelial adhesion molecules ICAM-1 and VCAM-1. Journal of Inflammation.

209. Miraj, S., & Alesaeidi, S. (2016). A systematic review study of therapeutic effects of Matricaria recuitta chamomile (chamomile). Electron Physician, 8(9): 3024–3031. Published online: 20 September 2016. doi: 10.19082/3024.

210. Wu, Y., Xu, Y., & Yao, L. (2011). Anti-inflammatory and Anti-allergic Effects of German Chamomile (Matricaria chamomilla L.). Journal of Essential Oil Bearing Plants, 14(5): 549–558. Received: 9 July 2010. Accepted: 22 February 2011, Published online: 12 March 2013.

211. Carretero, M. I., Gomes, C. S. F., & Tateo, F. Handbook of clay science. Edited by F. Bergaya, B.K.G. Theng and G. Lagaly. Elsevier Ltd. Chapter 11.5. Clays and Human Health. Developments in clay science. 2006; 1.

212. Williams, L. B., & Haydel, S. E. (2010). Evaluation of the medicinal use of clay minerals as antibacterial agents. *Int Geol Rev.* Author manuscript; available in PMC: 1 July 2011. Published in final edited form as: *Int Geol Rev. 52*(7/8): 745–770.

213. Charrie, J. C. *ABC de l'argile.* Grancher, Paris, 2007. ISBN 978-2-7339-1003-0.

214. Ahmed, S. H., Guillem, K., & Vandaele, Y. (2013). Sugar addiction: pushing the drug-sugar analogy to the limit. *Curr Opin Clin Nutr Metab Care. 16*(4): 434–439.

215. Wiss, D. A., Avena, N., & Rada, P. Sugar addiction: From evolution to revolution. *Front Psychiatry, 9*: 545. Published online: 7 November 2018.

216. DiNicolantonio, J. J., O'Keefe, J. H., & Wilson, W. L. Sugar addiction: is it real? A narrative review. *British Journal of Sports Science, 52*(14).

217. Pruimboom, L., & de Punder, K. (2015). The opioid effects of gluten exorphins: asymptomatic celiac disease. *J Health Popul Nutr, 33*: 24. Published online: 24 November 2015.

218. Teschemacher, H., Koch, G., & Brantl, V. (1997). Milk protein-derived opioid receptor ligands. *Biopolymers, 43*(2): 99–117.

219. Interview with Dr Natasha Campbell McBride.

220. Tabibian, N., Swehli, E., Boyd, A., Umbreen, A., & Tabibianb, J. H. (2017). Abdominal adhesions: A practical review of an often overlooked entity. *Ann Med Surg (Lond), 15*: 9–13. Published online: 31 January 2017.

221. van Steensel, S., van den Hil, L. C. L., Schreinemacher, M. H. F., ten Broek, R. P. G., van Goor, H., & Bouvy, N. D. *PLOS One.* Adhesion awareness in 2016: An update of the national survey of surgeons. Published: 17 August 2018. doi: 10.1371/journal.pone.0202418.

222. Rice, A. D., King, R., Reed, E. D., Patterson, K., Wurn, B. F. & Wurn, L. J. (2013). Manual physical therapy for non-surgical. Treatment of adhesion-related small bowel obstructions: Two case reports. *J Clin Med, 2*(1): 1–12.

223. Interview with Amanda Oswald.

224. Interview with Marty Ryan.

225. Interview with Isabel Spradlin.

226. Krebs, S., Omer, T. N., & Omer, B. (2010). Wormwood (Artemisia absinthium) suppresses tumour necrosis factor alpha and accelerates healing in patients with Crohn's disease—A controlled clinical trial. *Phytomedicine, 17*(5): 305–309. E-pub: 3 December 2009. doi: 10.1016/j.phymed.2009.10.013.

227. Omer, B., Krebs, S., Omer, H., & Noor. T. O. (2007). *Phytomedicine, 14*(2–3): 87–95. E-pub: 19 January 2007. Steroid-sparing effect of wormwood (Artemisia absinthium) in Crohn's disease: a double-blind placebo-controlled study.

228. Adesso, S., Russo, R., Quaroni, A., Autore G., & Marzocco, S. (2018). Astragalus membranaceus extract attenuates inflammation and oxidative stress in intestinal epithelial cells via NF-κB activation and Nrf2 response. *International Journal of Molecular Science, 19*(3): 800. https://doi.org/10.3390/ijms19030800.

229. Gerner-Rasmussen, J., Donatsky, A. M., & Bjerrum, F. (2018). The role of non-invasive imaging techniques in detecting intra-abdominal adhesions: a systematic review. *Langenbecks Arch Surg,* doi: 10.1007/s00423-018-1732-8.

BIBLIOGRAPHY

1. Sherwin, R. S., & Saccà, L. (1984). Effect of epinephrine on glucose metabolism in humans: contribution of the liver. *Am J Physiol, 247*(2 Pt 1): E157–165.
2. Porte, D. Jr., & Williams, R. H. (1966). Inhibition of insulin release by norepinephrine in man. *Science, 152*(3726): 1248–1250.
3. Macko, A. R., Yates, D. T., Chen, X., & Green, A. S. (2013). Elevated plasma norepinephrine inhibits insulin secretion, but adrenergic blockade reveals enhanced β-cell responsiveness in an ovine model of placental insufficiency at 0.7 of gestation. 4(5): 402–410.
4. Jutel, M., Akdis, M., & Akdis, C. A. (2009). Histamine, histamine receptors and their role in immune pathology. *Clin Exp Allergy, 39*(12): 1786–1800.
5. O'Mahony, L., Akdis, M., & Akdis, C. A. (2011). Regulation of the immune response and inflammation by histamine and histamine receptors. Swiss Institute of Allergy and Asthma Research (SIAF), University of Zurich, Davos, Switzerland. *128*(6): 1153–1162.
6. Rocha, S. M., Pires, J., Esteves, M., Graç, B., & Bernardino, L. (2014). Histamine: a new immunomodulatory player in the neuron-glia crosstalk. *Front Cell Neurosci, 8*: 120. Published online: 30 April 2014.
7. Hu, W. W., & Chen, Z. (2012). Role of Histamine and Its Receptors in Cerebral Ischemia. *ACS Chem Neurosci, 3*(4): 238–247.
8. Dunn, A. J., & Welch, J. (1991). Stress- and endotoxin-induced increases in brain tryptophan and serotonin metabolism depend on sympathetic nervous system activity. *J Neurochem, 57*(5): 1615–1622.
9. Johnson, E. W., Hughes, T. K. Jr., & Smith, E. M. (2005). ACTH enhancement of T-lymphocyte cytotoxic responses. Cell Mol Neurobiol, 25(3–4): 743–757.
10. Gatti, G. Cavallo, R., Sartori, M. L., del Ponte, D., Masera, R., Salvadori, A., Carignola, R., & Angeli, A. (1987). Inhibition by cortisol of human natural killer (NK) cell activity. *J Steroid Biochem, 26*(1): 49–58.

11. Raff, H., Sharma, S. T., & Nieman, L. K. (2014). Physiological basis for the etiology, diagnosis, and treatment of adrenal disorders: Cushing's Syndrome, adrenal insufficiency, and congenital adrenal hyperplasia, Compr Physiol, 4(2): 739–769.

12. Bertagna, X. (2017). Effects of chronic ACTH excess on human adrenal cortex. Front Endocrinol (Lausanne), 8: 43. Published online 8 March 2017. doi: 10.3389/fendo.2017.00043.

13. Donoho, C. J., Weigensberg, M. J., Adar Emken, B., Hsu, J. W., & Spruijt-Metz, D. (2011). Stress and abdominal fat: Preliminary evidence of moderation by the cortisol awakening response in Hispanic peripubertal girls. Obesity (Silver Spring), 19(5): 946–952.

14. Jeanrenaud, B. (1967). Effect of glucocorticoid hormones on fatty acid mobilization and re-esterification in rat adipose tissue. Biochem J, 103(3): 627–633.

15. Seck-Gassama, Ndoye, O., Mbodj, M., Akala, A., Cisse, F., Niang, M., & Ndoye, R. (2000). Serum cortisol level variations in thyroid diseases. Dakar Med, 45(1): 30–33.

16. Lin, C. H., Shih, T. H., Liu, S. T., Hsu, H. H., & Hwang, P. P. (2015). Cortisol regulates acid secretion of H^+-ATPase-rich Ionocytes in zebrafish (Danio rerio) embryos. Front Physiol, 6: 328. Published online: 17 November 2015. doi: 10.3389/fphys.2015.00328.

17. Seino, S., Seino, Y., Matsukura, S., Kurahachi, H., Ikeda, M., Yawata, M., & Imura, H. (1978). Effect of glucocorticoids on gastrin secretion in man. Gut, 19(1): 10–13. doi: 10.1136/gut.19.1.10.

18. Feuerstein, T. J., Gleichauf, O., & Landwehrmeyer, G. B. (1996). Modulation of cortical acetylcholine release by serotonin: the role of substance P interneurons. Naunyn Schmiedebergs Arch Pharmacol, 354(5): 618–626.

19. Pompili, M., Serafini, G., Innamorati, M., Möller-Leimkühler, A. M., Giupponi, G., Girardi, P., Tatarelli, R., & Lester, D. (2010). The hypothalamic-pituitary-adrenal axis and serotonin abnormalities: a selective overview of the implications of suicide prevention. Eur Arch Psychiatry Clin Neurosci, 260(8): 583–600. E-pub: 20 February 2010. doi: 10.1007/s00406-010-0108-z.

20. Walter, K. N., Corwin, E. J., Ulbrecht, J., Demers, L. M., Bennett, J. M., Whetzel, C. A., & Klein, L. C. (2012). Elevated thyroid stimulating hormone is associated with elevated cortisol in healthy young men and women. Biomed Central, Thyroid Research, 5: 13. Published online: 30 October 2012. doi: 10.1186/1756-6614-5-13.

21. Mohammad, I., Starskaia, I., Nagy, T., Guo, J., Yatkin, E., Väänänen, K., Watford, W. T., Chen, Z. (2018). Estrogen receptor α contributes to T-cell-mediated autoimmune inflammation by promoting T-cell activation and proliferation. Sci Signal, 11(526). pii: eaap9415. doi: 10.1126/scisignal.aap9415.

22. Cutolo, M., Capellino, S., Sulli, A., Serioli, B., Secchi, M. E., Villaggio, B., & Straub, R. H. (2006). Estrogens and autoimmune diseases. Ann N Y Acad Sci, 1089: 538–547.

23. El-Tawil, A. M. (2008). Oestrogens and Crohn's disease: the missed link. Andrologia, 40(3): 1415. doi: 10.1111/j.1439-0272.2008.00836.x.

24. Mauvais-Jarvis, F., Clegg, D. J., & Hevener, A. L. (2013). The role of estrogens in control of energy balance and glucose homeostasis. Endocr Rev, 34(3): 309–338.

25. Santin, A. P., & Furlanetto, T. W. (2011). Role of Estrogen in Thyroid Function and Growth Regulation. J Thyroid Res, 2011: 875125. Published online 2011 May 4. doi: 10.4061/2011/875125.

26. Gupta, P., Agarwal, A., Gupta, V., Singh, P. K., Pantola, C., & Amit, S. (2012). Expression and clinicopathological significance of estrogen and progesterone receptors in gallbladder cancer. *Gastrointest Cancer Res*, 5(2): 41–47.

27. Nagelkerken, L. (1998). Role of Th1 and Th2 cells in autoimmune demyelinating disease. Brazilian Journal of Medical and Biological Research. *31*(1): 55–60.

28. Graham, J. D., & Clarke, C. L. (1997). Physiological action of progesterone in target tissues. *Endocrine Reviews*, 18(4): 502–519.

29. Franco, J. S., Amaya-Amaya, J., & Anaya, J. M. Autoimmunity from bench to bedside. Chapter 30. Thyroid disease and autoimmune diseases. Bogota (Colombia): El Rosario University Press; 18 July 2013. ISBN-13: 9789587383669 (paper) ISBN-13: 9789587383768 (digital).

30. Hoermann, R., Eckl, W., Hoermann, C., & Larisch, R. (2010). Complex relationship between free thyroxine and TSH in the regulation of thyroid function. *Eur J Endocrinol*, 162(6): 1123–1129. E-pub: 18 March 2010. doi: 10.1530/EJE-10-0106.

31. Sinha, R., & Yen, P. M. Endotext. Cellular action of thyroid hormone. Last Update: 20: June 2018.

32. Ohashi, H., & Itoh, M. (1994). Effects of thyroid hormones on the lymphocyte phenotypes in rats: changes in lymphocyte subsets related to thyroid function. *Endocr Regul*, 28(3): 117–123.

33. Watanabe, K., Iwatani, Y., Hidaka, Y., Watanabe, M., & Amino, N. (1995). Long-term effects of thyroid hormone on lymphocyte subsets in spleens and thymuses of mice. *Endocr J*, 42(5): 661–668.

34. Gullo, L., Pezzilli, R., Bellanova, B., D'ambrosi, A., Alvisi, V., & Barbara, L. (1991). Influence of the thyroid on exocrine pancreatic function. Unit for the Study of Pancreatic Disease, Institute of Medicine. *Gastroenterology*, 100: 1392–1396.

35. Isaac, R., Boura-Halfon, S., Gurevitch, D., Shainskaya, A., Levkovitz Y., & Zick, Y. Selective serotonin reuptake inhibitors (SSRIs) inhibit insulin secretion and action in pancreatic beta cells. Journal of biological chemistry.

36. Leal-Cerro, A., Povedano, J., Astorga, R., Gonzalez, M., Silva, H., Garcia-Pesquera, F., Casanueva, F. F., & Dieguez, C. (1999). The growth hormone (GH)-releasing hormone-GH-insulin-like growth factor-1 axis in patients with fibromyalgia syndrome. *J Clin Endocrinol Metab*, 84(9): 3378–3381.

37. Hussain, M. A., Schmitz, O., Mengel, A., Glatz, Y., Christiansen, J. S., Zapf, J., & Froesch, E. R. (1994). Comparison of the effects of growth hormone and insulin-like growth factor I on substrate oxidation and on insulin sensitivity in growth hormone-deficient humans. *J Clin Invest*, 94(3): 1126–1133.

38. Wang, T., Lu, J., Xu, Y., Li, M., Sun, J., Zhang, J., i Xu, B., Xu, M., Chen, Y., Bi, Y., Wang, W., & Ning, G. (2013). Circulating prolactin associates with diabetes and impaired glucose regulation. A population-based study. PhD Diabetes Care, 36(7): 1974–1980. Published online: 12 June 2013. doi: 10.2337/dc12-1893.

39. Müller, M. J., von Schütz, B., Huhnt, H. J., Zick, R., Mitzkat, H. J., von zur Mühlen A. (1986). Glucoregulatory function of thyroid hormones: interaction with insulin depends on the prevailing glucose concentration. *J Clin Endocrinol Metab*, 63(1): 62–71.

40. Lyte, M. Pearls. Microbial endocrinology in the microbiome-gut-brain axis: How bacterial production and utilization of neurochemicals influence behaviour. Published: 14 November 2013.

41. Lyte, M. (2011). Probiotics function mechanistically as delivery vehicles for neuroactive compounds: Microbial endocrinology in the design and use of probiotics. *Bioessays*, *33*(8): 574–581. E-pub: 6 July 2011.

42. Peyrin-Biroulet, L., Loftus, E. V., Colombel, J., & Sandborn, W. J. (2010). The natural history of adult Crohn's disease in population-based cohorts. *Am J Gastroenterol*, *105*: 289–297. doi: 10.1038/ajg.2009.579.

43. Beaugerie, L., Seksik, P., Nion-Larmurier, I., Gendre, J., & Cosnes, J. Predictors of Crohn's disease. *Gastroenterology*, *130*: 650–656. doi: 10.1053/j.gastro.2005.12.019.

44. Mafra, D., Lobo, J. C., Barros, A. F., Koppe, L., Vaziri, N. D., & Fouque, D. (2014). Role of altered intestinal microbiota in systemic inflammation and cardiovascular disease in chronic kidney disease. *Future Microbiol*, *9*(3): 399–410. doi: 10.2217/fmb.13.165.

45. Herrera, A. J., Espinosa-Oliva, A. M., Carrillo-Jiménez, A., Oliva-Martín, M. J., García-Revilla, J., García-Quintanilla, A., de Pablos, R. M., & Venero, K. L. (2015). Relevance of chronic stress and the two faces of microglia in Parkinson's disease. *Front Cell Neurosci*, *9*: 312. Published online: 14 August 2015.

46. Buckley, A., & Turner, J. R. (2018). Cell biology of tight junction barrier regulation and mucosal disease. Cold Spring Harb Perspect Biol, *10*(1).

47. Franke, A., McGovern Dermot, P. B., Barrett, J. C., Wang, K., Radford-Smith, G. L., Ahmad, T., Lees, V. W., Balschun, T., Lee, J., Roberts, R., Anderson, C. A., Bis, J. C., Bumpstead, S., Ellinghaus, D., Festen, E. M., Georges, M., Green, T., Haritunians, T., Jostins, L., Latiano, A., Mathew, C. G., Montgomery, G. W., Prescott, N. J., Raychaudhuri, S., Rotter, J. I., Schumm, P., Sharma, Y., Simms, L. A., Taylor, K. D., & Whiteman, D., et al. (2010). Genome-wide meta-analysis increases to 71 the number of confirmed Crohn's disease susceptibility loci. *Nat Genet*, *42*: 1118–1125. doi: 10.1038/ng.717.

48. Van Limbergen, J., Radford-Smith, G., & Satsangi, J. (2014). Advances in IBD genetics. *Nat Rev Gastroenterol Hepatol*, *11*: 372–385. doi: 10.1038/nrgastro.2014.27.

49. Hunt, K. A., Mistry, V., Bockett, N. A., Ahmad, T., Ban, M., Barker, J. N., Barrett, J. C., Blackburn, H., Brand, O., Burren, O., Capon, F., Compston, A., Gough Stephen, C. L., Jostins, L., Kong, Y., Lee, J. C., Lek, M., MacArthur, D. G., Mansfield, J. C., Mathew, C. G., Mein, C. A., Mirza, M., Nutland, S., Onengut-Gumuscu, S., Papouli, E., Parkes, M., Rich, S. S., Sawcer, S., Satsangi, J., & Simmonds, M. J., et al. (2013). Negligible impact of rare autoimmune-locus coding-region variants on missing heritability. *Nature*, *498*: 232–235. doi: 10.1038/nature12170.

50. Ventham, N. T., Kennedy, N. A., Nimmo, E. R., & Satsangi, J. (2013). Beyond gene discovery in inflammatory bowel disease: the emerging role of epigenetics. *Gastroenterology*, *145*: 293–308. doi: 10.1053/j.gastro.2013.05.050.

51. Heghes, S. C., Vostinaru, O., Rus, L. M., Mogosan, C., Adela Luga, C., & Filip, L. (2019). Francesca Mancianti, Academic Editor Antispasmodic effect of essential oils and their constituents: A review. *Molecules*, *24*(9): 1675. Published online: 29 April 2019. doi: 10.3390/molecules24091675.

52. Alammar, N., Wang, L., Saberi, B., Nanavati, J., Holtmann, G., Shinohara, R. T., & Mullin, G. E. (2019). The impact of peppermint oil on the irritable bowel syndrome: a meta-analysis of the pooled clinical data. *BMC Complement Altern Med*, *19*: 21. Published online: 17 January 2019. doi: 10.1186/s12906-018-2409-0.

53. Williams, L. B., Haydel, S. E., Giese, R. F. Jr., & Eberl, D. D. (2008). Chemical and mineralogical characteristics of French green clays used for healing. Clays Clay Miner.

Author manuscript; available in PMC: 10 December 2008. Published in final edited form as: Clays Clay Miner, *56*(4): 437–452.

54. Williams, L. B., & Haydel, S. E. (2010). Evaluation of the medicinal use of clay minerals as antibacterial agents. *Int Geol Rev*. Author manuscript; available in PMC: 1 July 2011. Published in final edited form as: *Int Geol Rev, 52*(7/8): 745–770.

55. Williams, L. B., Metge, D. W., Eberl, D. D., Harvey, R. W., Turner, A. G., Prapaipong, P., & Poret-Peterson, A. T. (2011). What makes a natural clay antibacterial? Environ Sci Technol. Author manuscript; available in PMC: 29 June 2011. Published in final edited form as: *Environ Sci Technol, 45*(8): 3768–3773. Published online: 17 March 2011. doi: 10.1021/es1040688.

56. Ising, M., Ising, M., Max Planck Institute of Psychiatry, Munich, Germany; Holsboer, F. (2006). Genetics of stress response and stress-related disorders. *Dialogues Clin Neurosci, 8*(4): 433–444.

57. Ellis, H., Moran, B. J., Thompson, J. N., Parker, M. C., Wilson, M. S., Menzies, D., McGuire, A., Lower, A. M., Hawthorn, R. J., O'Brien, F., Buchan, S., & Crowe, A. M. (1999). Adhesion-related hospital readmissions after abdominal and pelvic surgery: a retrospective cohort study. *Lancet, 353*(9163): 1476–1480.

58. Stommel, M. W. J., Schipper, L. J., van Goor, H., & ten Broek Langenbecks R. P. G. (2016). Risk factors for future repeat abdominal surgery. Chema Strik, corresponding author. Arch Surg, *401*(6): 829–837. Published online: 13 April 2016.

59. ten Broek, R. P. G., Issa, Y., van Santbrink, E. V. P., Bouvy, N. D., Kruitwagen, R. F. M., Jeekel, J., Bakkum, E. A., Rovers, M. M., & van Goor, H. (2013). Burden of adhesions in abdominal and pelvic surgery: systematic review and meta-analysis. *BMJ*, 347 doi: https://doi.org/10.1136/bmj.f5588 (Published: 3 October 2013). Cite this as: BMJ, 2013; 347:f5588.

60. Moeller, S., Lücke, C., Heinen, C., Bewernick, B. H., Aydin, M., Lam, A. P., Grömer, T. W., Philipsen, A., & Müller, H. H. O. (2019). Vagus nerve stimulation as an adjunctive neurostimulation tool in treatment-resistant depression. *J Vis Exp*, (143). doi: 10.3791/58264.

61. Ma, P., Yu, P., Yu, J., Wang, W., Ding, Y., Chen, C., Chen, X., Zhao, K., Zuo, T., He, X., Shi, Q., & Ren, J. (2016). Effects of Nicotine and Vagus Nerve in Severe Acute Pancreatitis-Associated Lung Injury in Rats. *Pancreas, 45*(4): 552–560. doi: 10.1097/MPA.0000000000000575.

62. Jiang, W. D., Zhou, X. Q., Zhang, L., Liu, Y., Wu, P., Jiang, J., Kuang, S.Y., Tang, L., Tang, W. N., Zhang, Y. A., Shi, H. Q., and Feng, L. (2019). Vitamin A deficiency impairs intestinal physical barrier function of fish. Fish Shellfish Immunol,. pii: S1050-4648(19)30072-5. E-pub ahead of print. doi: 10.1016/j.fsi.2019.01.056.

63. Wilkinson-Smith, V., Dellschaft, N., Ansell, J., Hoad, C., Marciani, L., Gowland, P., & Spiller, R. (2019). Aliment Pharmacol Ther, doi: 10.1111/apt.15127. [Epub ahead of print] Mechanisms underlying effects of kiwifruit on intestinal function shown by MRI in healthy volunteers.

64. Vinokurova, L. V., Baimakanova, G. E.,. Krasovsky, S. A., Silvestrova, S. Y., Dubtsova, E. A., Varvanina, G. G., & Bordin, D. S. (2018). Functional insufficiency of the pancreas and the metabolic activity of the microbiota in cystic fibrosis adults patients. Ter Arkh, *90*(10): 84–88. doi: 10.26442/terarkh2018901084-88.

65. Kusakabe, J., Anderson, B., Liu, J., Williams, G. A., Chapman, W. C., Doyle, M. M. B., Khan, A. S., Sanford, D. E., Hammill, C. W., Strasberg, S. M., Hawkins, W. G., & Fields,

R. C. (2019). Long-term endocrine and exocrine insufficiency after pancreatectomy. J Gastrointest Surg, doi: 10.1007/s11605-018-04084-x.

66. Quigley, E. M. M. The spectrum of small intestinal bacterial overgrowth. *Curr Gastroenterol Rep, 21*(1):3. doi: 10.1007/s11894-019-0671-z. (SIBO). Gastroenterology, 1 February 2019. pii: S0016-5085(19)30352-X. doi: 10.1053/j.gastro.2018.12.043.

67. Stancill, J. S., Broniowska, K. A., Oleson, B. J. Naatz, A., Corbett, J. A., Uc, A., & Husain, S. Z. (2019). Pancreatitis in children. Pancreatic β-cells detoxify H_2O_2 through the peroxiredoxin/thioredoxin antioxidant system. *J Biol Chem*, pii: jbc.RA118.006219. doi: 10.1074/jbc.RA118.006219.

68. Boelen, A., Kwakkel, J., & Fliers, E. (2011). Beyond low plasma T3: Local thyroid hormone metabolism during inflammation and infection. *Endocrine Reviews, 32*(5): 670–693.

69. Zoccali, C., Tripepi, G., Cutrupi, S., Pizzini, P., & Mallamaci, F. (2005). Low triiodothyronine: A new facet of inflammation in end-stage renal disease. *J Am Soc Nephrol, 16*: 2789–2795.

70. Shizuma, T. Concomitant thyroid disorders and inflammatory bowel disease: A literature review. Hindawi Publishing Corporation BioMed Research International 2016; Article ID 5187061: 12.

71. Bianchi, G., Marchesini, G., Zoli, M., Falasconi, M. C., Lervese, T., Vecchi, F., & Magalotti, D. S. (1993). Clinical Rheumatology. Thyroid involvement in chronic inflammatory rheumatological disorders. *12*(4): 479–484.

72. Ruggieri, A., Gagliardi, M. C., & Anticoli, S. (2018). Sex-dependent outcome of hepatitis B and C viruses infections: Synergy of sex hormones and immune responses? Front Immunol.

73. Moulton, V. R. (2018). Sex Hormones in Acquired Immunity and Autoimmune Disease. Front Immunol.

74. Gubbels Bupp, M. R., Potluri, T., Fink, A. L., & Klein, S. L. (2018). The confluence of sex hormones and aging on immunity. Front Immunol.

75. Dupuis, M. L., Conti, F., Maselli, A., Pagano, M. T., Ruggieri, A., Anticoli, S., Fragale, A., Gabriele, L., Gagliardi, M. C., Sanchez, M., Ceccarelli, F., Alessandri, C., Valesini, G., Ortona, E., & Pierdominici, M. (2018). The Natural agonist of estrogen receptor β silibinin plays an immunosuppressive role representing a potential therapeutic tool in rheumatoid arthritis. Front Immunol.

76. Kharrazian, D. The Potential Roles of Bisphenol A (BPA) Pathogenesis in Autoimmunity. Hindawi Publishing Corporation Autoimmune Diseases Volume 2014, Article ID 743616, 12 pages. http://dx.doi.org/10.1155/2014/743616.

77. Morales, L. B. J., Loo, K., Liu, H. B., Peterson, Tiwari-Woodruff, S., & Voskuhl, R. R. (2006). Neurobiology of disease. Treatment with an estrogen receptor ligand. Is neuroprotective in experimental autoimmune encephalomyelitis. *The Journal of Neuroscience, 26*(25): 6823–6833.

78. Dragin, N., Nancy, P., Villegas, J., Roussin, R., Panse, R. L., & Berrih-Aknin, S. (2017). Balance between Estrogens and Proinflammatory Cytokines Regulates Chemokine Production Involved in Thymic Germinal Center Formatio. Scientific Reports.

79. Zadeh, A. R., Ghadimi, K., Mohammadi, B., Hatamian, H., Naghibi, S. N., & Danaeiniya, A. Effects of estrogen and progesterone on different immune cells related to multiple sclerosis. Caspian Journal of Neurological Sciences *'Caspian J Neurol Sci' 4*(2): 13.

80. Crider A., & Pillai, A. Estrogen signaling as a therapeutic target in neurodevelopmental disorders. *J Pharmacol Exp Ther, 360*: 48–58.

INDEX

Paul Michael BA, BSc, MCPP
www.endobiogenicmedicine.co.uk